MANUAL MEDICINE FOR THE PRIMARY CARE TEAM: A HANDS-ON APPROACH

MANUAL MEDICINE FOR THE PRIMARY CARE TEAM: A HANDS-ON APPROACH

Frank J. Domino, MD

Professor
University of Massachusetts Medical School
Dept. of Family Medicine and Community Health
Worcester, Massachusetts

Steve Messineo, DPT

Owner and Executive Director
All-Access Physical Therapy
Shrewsbury, Massachusetts

Mark Powicki, DPT

Owner and Executive Director
All-Access Physical Therapy
Shrewsbury, Massachusetts

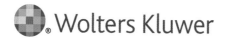

Philadelphia • Baltimore • New York • London
Buenos Aires • Hong Kong • Sydney • Tokyo

Executive Editor: Rebecca Gaertner
Product Development Editor: Liz Schaeffer
Editorial Coordinator: Emily Buccieri
Marketing Manager: Rachel Mante Leung
Senior Production Project Manager: Alicia Jackson
Design Coordinator: Holly McLaughlin
Senior Manufacturing Coordinator: Beth Welsh
Prepress Vendor: TNQ Technologies

9 8 7 6 5 4 3 2 1

Printed in China

Library of Congress Cataloging-in-Publication Data

ISBN-13: 978-1-9751-1147-2

Cataloging in Publication data available on request from publisher

shop.lww.com

DEDICATION & ACKNOWLEDGMENTS

To my wife Darcy who has always been my biggest supporter as a physical therapist, practice owner, and entrepreneur, no matter how "hairbrained" some of my ideas have been. And to my wonderful children—Nick, Zach, and Maddy. You are my inspiration; I am incredibly grateful to have been blessed with such a wonderful family. My Mom, Dad, and brother Mike—thank you for your love and guidance throughout my life. And to my two partners in this endeavor, Frank Domino, MD and Mark Powicki, DPT. Without their shared knowledge and passion for helping people, this book would never have been written.

—Steve Messineo

To my wife Sandra, thank you for your unwavering love and support. Your love makes me feel like a super hero! You motivate and inspire me to become the best version of "me." My son Brendan is the greatest gift I could ever ask for; you taught me how to love. I hope I have provided you with a solid foundation to become your own man, one of love, honesty, integrity, and discipline while maintaining a grateful, humble heart. And to my parents: Kate and Ed. Thank you for loving me unconditionally and providing me with every opportunity to be successful! I am truly blessed and grateful to have such amazing parents! To Steve Messineo, my friend and business partner. Without your marketing prowess and drive we would only have a "Field of Dreams." And to Frank Domino, MD, for your vision and trust; your caring and compassion to make a difference in the lives of your patients is truly inspiring!

—Mark Powicki

Healing by touch is not part of the typical allopathic training; I thank my friends Vasilos (Bill) Chrisostomidis, DO, and Mark Steenbergen, DO, who introduced and reinforced the benefits of hands-on care, and to my two coauthors Steve Messineo and Mark Powicki, who helped me heal after countless breakdowns in my physical well-being. And to my family; my parents, Jean and Frank, my wife, Sylvia, and daughter, Molly, for their love and support.

—Frank J. Domino

We hope every clinician who reads this book finds the treatment techniques to be of great value to their patients. We would like to thank all who have put their trust in our services for their patients over the years. This includes Frank Domino, Joe Daigneault, Lee Mancini, J. Herb Stevenson, Vasilos (Bill) Chrisostomidis, Brian Busconi, Nicola DeAngelis, Michael Brown, Steve Desio, Ingrid Fuller, Phil Lahey, Jr, Daniel Freitas, Michael Burdulis, Mary Kay O'Connor-Seguin, Richard Orino, Ken Stevens, David Mazin, Chris Vinton, Kathleen Mitchell, James Narius, Raymond Zhou, Paul Pongor, Jerrianne Seger, Michael Reyes, John Stevenson, Mary O'Brien, John McCahan, Atreyi Chakrabarti, Danuta Antkowiak, and Jay Broadhurst.

To the incredible staff of All-Access Physical Therapy, especially Pam Powell, Patti Moore, Karen Girard, Julia Salas, Jill Trovo, and Alexander Stech. They and the rest of our staff make our jobs as practice owners extremely easy; we are truly grateful for their dedication and support.

This book is the result of countless hours of effort from our wonderful team at Wolters Kluwer, Inc.

To Elizabeth Schaeffer, Emily Buccieri, Sharon Zinner, and Rebecca Gaertner; this book and video was a new adventure for us all; thank you for your vision and patience.

And for the openness and ingenuity of the team at Pri-Med, Inc., who supported our hope to share this knowledge with clinicians throughout the country. This includes Sara Floros, Cameron Milkiewicz, Rick Watson, and their entire team. And to Marijo "MJ" Adamcik and the folks at Rock Tape, Inc. for their generous support of our live programs.

At the University of Massachusetts Medical School, thanks to Karen Rayla, Maryanne Adams, Jennifer Masoud, Mary Lindholm, and Dan Lasser. And especially to Robert Baldor, for his wisdom, mentorship, and patience in the pursuit of this book.

The authors would also like to acknowledge the contributions of Terri Ann Joy, Director of Operations, for Encounter TeleHealth, for consulting on the billing and coding sections of this text.

CONTENTS

PART I • OVERVIEW OF MANUAL MEDICINE   1

1   Introduction   2

2   What Is Manual Medicine?   4

3   Mindfulness and Breathing   7

4   Kinesiology Tape   9

5   Coding And Billing For Manual Medicine   11

PART II • TREATMENTS   15

6   Neck and Upper Back Pain   16

7   Shoulder   50

8   Acute Chest Discomfort   71

9   Arm, Elbow, and Wrist Pain   93

10   Acute Low Back Pain   119

11   Upper Leg And Hip   152

12   Knee Pain   177

13   Foot and Ankle Pain   202

Index   229

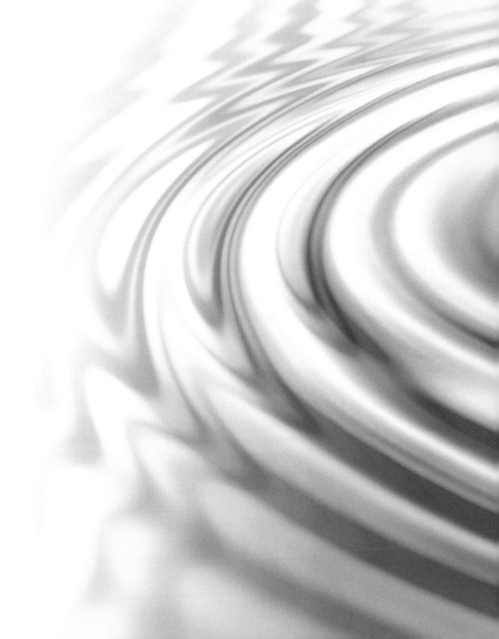

PART | 1

OVERVIEW OF MANUAL MEDICINE

CHAPTER | 1

INTRODUCTION

Long before medications and surgery became the standard treatments in health care, the laying of hands on patients was used to relieve pain and improve patient care. When you are ill, it feels good to be in "the hands" of a caregiver. If the patient presenting to you is in pain, the ability to quickly and safely address that pain in the office is gratifying for the patient and satisfying to the clinician. Physical therapists, osteopaths, massage therapists, and acupuncturists have long known this gratification.

Allopathic providers (those trained to treat disease with primarily medication and surgery) are taught to focus their care of musculoskeletal disorders by writing prescriptions, often for pain medications, and making referrals to orthopedic surgery and/or physical therapy. Osteopathic providers in the United States, however, are trained to use their hands to help patients heal in addition to the methods of allopathic providers (to use medicine and surgery).

This emphasis of drugs and surgery may have led to unintentional harm. Medication overutilization has played a large role in today's opioid crisis and the increase in resistant infections such as methicillin-resistant *Staphylococcus aureus*.

Orthopedic surgeons are trained to solve problems with surgery. Yet, in the past 5 years, the surgery used to treat back pain (spinal fusion) has been found to be no better than nonsurgical methods; likewise, knee (meniscus injury) and shoulder surgery for impingement syndrome (rotator cuff tendonitis) and osteoarthritis may be no better than conservative care (rehabilitation through physical therapy). Unfortunately, conservative approaches are underutilized owing to inconsistencies in insurance coverage and patient hesitation regarding their benefits.

This book will expand your care of patients with musculoskeletal complaints. In doing so, you will lower the risk of unnecessary surgery and potentially harmful medication.

When you physically engage a patient, and they feel better, you get professional satisfaction far beyond the prescription or referral. Injecting a shoulder for an acute impingement syndrome is one of the few interventions provided in the ambulatory setting by an allopathic provider which the patient receives rapid pain relief and the provider receives the sense of being the one to lessen the patient's suffering.

Manual medicine has the combined goal of helping patients quickly feel better while you as the provider get a sense that your "hands-on" care improved both in the moment relief of suffering and long-term clinical outcomes. It reinforces the benefit of treating their complaint with physical rehabilitation.

The goal of this book is to introduce a treatment approach to musculoskeletal complaints using manual techniques and proper referral. This will be accomplished via a "functional" rather than diagnostic physical examination. Written description and video demonstration of simple and effective maneuvers will be offered that anyone with medical training can provide. There is no additional malpractice risk, and using this approach will likely *lower* your liability because of fewer drug-drug interactions and adverse effects. Finally, most insurers will pay for your extra care, with appropriate billing and documentation discussed.

Manual medicine is a win-win, providing great benefit for your patients and for your professional satisfaction.

C H A P T E R | 2

WHAT IS MANUAL MEDICINE?

The origins of manual medicine begin in the worlds of physical therapy and osteopathy. Both realms have long recognized many musculoskeletal complaints and other clinical syndromes can extend from anatomic dysfunction. Headaches and hypertension are two examples where improper muscle tone can lead to symptoms, poor posture and breathing habits and ultimately into diagnoses allopathic medicine treats with "a pill." Allopathic medicine may suggest exercise or stress reduction, but in almost every case, these two conditions are primarily addressed with an oral agent.

Manual medicine focuses diagnosis on regions that are working in a less optimal way and tries to correct that dysfunction. One treatment with manual medicine does not "cure" anything, but for many acute and chronic ailments, it can provide a path to decreased and ultimately no symptoms.

For the sake of this book, manual medicine is defined as any hands-on method that helps treat acute and chronic musculoskeletal pain.

Approaches and Philosophies

Myofascial Release

This approach is based on the theory that the body's fasciae are interconnected. When the fascia of a particular area is dysfunctional, trigger points arise. Myofascial release is a massage technique that focuses on location and mobilization of these trigger points, which results in improved muscle function and decreased patient symptoms.

Positional Release Therapy

Dysfunction can lead to the formation of tender points (in muscles, ligaments, tendons, and joints). Treatment requires the clinician to:
• Identify the tender point through palpation,
• Maintain pressure on the tender point while you passively move the patient's body toward the position of greatest comfort (resolving the tender point);
• Hold the patient in this position for an extended period (often a minimum of 90 seconds);
• Passively return the body part to neutral, resulting in the dissolution of the tender point.

Muscle Energy Techniques

Muscles that are shortened and in spasm can be lengthened by treating these muscles or by treating their antagonists. The treatment involves moving the region to its limit (called a restrictive barrier), then having the patient isometrically contract against a resistance, then relax. In that relaxation, move the region to a new limit and repeat. It has two approaches, post isometric relaxation (PIR) and reciprocal inhibition (RI).

Post Isometric Relaxation

Also called proprioceptive neuromuscular facilitation (PNF) or facilitated stretching, PIR is based on the concept that when a shortened, tight muscle isometrically contracts against a fixed resistance, and then relaxes, it will more easily lengthen. As the contraction relaxes, the muscle group can then be moved to a new limit and stretched again. This technique was first developed as a method of rehabilitating stroke victims. PNF will be the major focus of this book.

Reciprocal Inhibition

This approach uses the same technique as PIR, but here the painful and shortened muscle is moved to its limit and its antagonist muscles are isometrically contracted against resistance. As the antagonistic muscle group contracts, the painful muscle group naturally relaxes. It is most useful when the involved, painful muscle group is too painful to move.

Benefits of Manual Medicine

There are many and sometimes contradictory schools of thoughts on these techniques, and their best evidence in the medical literature is limited to small randomized controlled trials. Yet, the benefits of these techniques far outweigh their risks and, most importantly, support definitive care. As noted, manual medicine does not "cure" anything after one treatment. If a patient is suffering from a musculoskeletal complaint, providing an in-office treatment that reduces their symptoms may help them feel better and help them understand that more than "a pill" is needed to fix what ails them. It will also reinforce that definitive care comes from rehabilitation, most often through physical therapy.

Rehabilitation of what is injured and change in patient's behavior (often posture or work habits) are the keys to long-term recovery. Manual medicine provides the short-term relief and offers the patient a motivation that further physical maneuvers will make them feel and function better.

The application of manual medicine techniques requires proper patient placement, clear verbal commands, and the use of mindfulness-related diaphragmatic breathing. The next chapter will describe the role of mindfulness and breathing and its value in helping address muscle pain. A subsequent chapter addresses application of kinesiology tape to help sustain a patient's improved symptoms. Like the schools and theories of manual medicine, kinesiology tape has a large cohort of advocates but a limited literature base to support its use. Only small randomized controlled trials have been published demonstrating its benefit in pain control. Kinesiology tape's likely benefit is its supporting role to rehabilitation via physical therapy.

Methods and the Approach of This Book

Each chapter is based on symptoms location. This book's approach focuses on regions, rather than specific muscles, as little happens in the body to just one muscle. The process is the same as in all of medicine; a thorough history is obtained, generating a differential diagnosis. A physical examination refines that differential. Then treatment is initiated.

Treatment typically involves:

1. Identifying the short, tender muscle(s) to be treated
2. Moving that body part so those muscles are gently stretched to their limit ("end point")
3. Asking the patient to push against your resistance (most often, into your hands) with a gentle, 10% effort (isometric contraction)
4. Asking the patient to take three diaphragmatic "belly breaths" while sustaining this contraction, then relax
5. As the patient relaxes, moving the region to its new limit.
6. Repeating the treatment for three stretch-relax cycles

The success of this approach lies in the relaxation of a shortened, spasmed muscle following its isometric contraction. This simple process will result in patients having fewer symptoms and will expand their understanding that what is causing pain needs to be solved by addressing muscular dysfunction through rehabilitation.

Manual techniques are easily applied in the course of a brief office visit. It may include two to four techniques, teaching that patient to use diaphragmatic breathing, and possibly the application of kinesiology tape. Patient eduction exercises are also included for the patient to use while waiting to start physical therapy. It is that simple.

Your efforts are rewarded by the patient leaving your office feeling better and your ability to bill insurers for your efforts. Patients should leave understanding that, because of your efforts, their ultimate cure comes from a change in their exercise routine (via physical therapy) and, possibly, a change in how they go about their day, which may be causing their problem.

CHAPTER | 3
MINDFULNESS AND BREATHING

What is this chapter doing here? A book on manual medicine discussing mindfulness? Therapeutically, mindfulness and mindful breathing have a strong influence on both physical and mental outcomes. To effectively apply the techniques described in this book, you must help patients learn to mindfully breathe during treatment.

For example, try to move your head toward your shoulder without moving your clavicle. Which side seems less mobile? Then:

- grab that side of your head with your opposite hand (if the left neck seems more restricted, use your right hand) and gently pull your head away from the restricted side and toward the opposite shoulder to its end point;

- then, using 10% effort, try to move your head back to neutral against your hand;

- now, using your abdominal muscles to deepen each breath, take three deep breaths, then relax.

- Move your head again in the less mobile direction; does it move further now?

Hopefully you felt the effect of the deep breaths on the muscles in your neck. Mindful breaths, also called *belly* breaths, help facilitate a greater stretch than without the breaths. Many of the techniques outlined in this book include the use of these belly breaths.

Let us begin with a few definitions:

- **Meditation:** the practice of focusing and refocusing your attention on an activity (such as saying a mantra); it is an activity you intentionally do to center and calm the brain.

- **Mindfulness:** a type of meditation; an awareness of what is going on in your world, a deliberate attention to stimuli in your environment.

- **Mindful breathing:** using your abdominal muscles (rather than just the chest's intercostal muscles) to take a deep breath. This approach drops your diaphragm, increases lung volume and venous return to the heart, and contributes to a host of other physiologic parameters. It is a deliberate focus of your attention on an activity.

- **Method for mindful breathing:** Place one hand on your abdomen and the other on your chest. Attempt to take a deep breath by primarily expanding your abdomen. Your abdominal hand should move greatly, while the chest hand should move very little.

Learning mindful breathing has clinical benefits, including reducing stress, improving oxygen uptake, elevating mood, and improving athletic performance. Mindful breathing can be applied as the focus of a meditation, where you sit and pay attention to your breath. When your attention wanders (which is normal, and not a sign that you "cannot meditate"), you will eventually realize your mind has wandered and you then bring your focus back to your breath.

Mindful breathing can be applied as a therapeutic intervention, as in its use in manual medicine. It can be an excellent (and quick) stress reliever when tied to an image. The "One-Second Mindfulness" method is a simple and highly practical method as taught by Jay Winner, MD, author of *Relaxation on the Run*. To practice this technique, place an image of a place you find relaxing at various locations where stress may be common. I place a beach scene just above my computer's screen at my desk (the home of the stress-inducing electronic health record) and in the hallway leading to my examination rooms. When I see this beach scene, I stop and take one deep belly breath, then proceed. Doing so will lower your stress and focus your attention. Add this relaxation technique to a daily practice of meditation, and it is even more effective.

For more information on mindfulness and breathing, check out the Greater Good in Action website: https://ggia.berkeley.edu/practice/mindful_breathing. For more information on how to apply mindfulness into clinical practice, see Jay Winner's free website of resources: https://stressremedy.com/. I often recommend both websites to patients who wish to get a better handle on their response to stress.

CHAPTER | 4
KINESIOLOGY TAPE

Also called K-Taping and Kinesio Taping, the application of stretchy kinesiology tape over a damaged or injured muscle or muscles is increasingly used to help facilitate healing. This method was developed in the 1960s, and its mechanism of action is theorized as taping gently lifts the skin and attached tissues covering a muscle so that blood and lymph can move more freely around that muscle. Use of the tape further supports the injured region while it recovers and may provide an awareness of that region, making the wearer less apt to continue to injure it (Figure 4-1).

There is an evidence base to the use of kinesiology tape. Systematic review level data show its use has analgesic effect. This alone is of value because there is almost no risk to the tape's use (except potential irritant reaction to the adhesive), whereas even over-the-counter acetaminophen and nonsteroidal anti-inflammatory drugs have potential risks and interactions. Additional studies have shown kinesiology tape's efficacy by body region, with successful use in the upper back and neck, shoulder and elbow, and lower back, and in syndromes such as carpal tunnel and lymphedema.

However, these are small randomized controlled trials showing mixed results. For example, there may be physiologic improvement but not always patient-oriented outcomes. Other trials have shown symptom-based improvements without clearly demonstrated physiologic benefit.

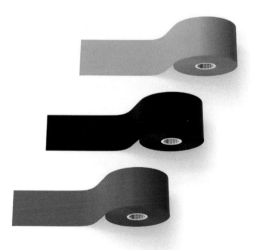

Figure 4-1 • Kinesiology tape. (Photo courtesy of RockTape.)

Taping Methods

Kinesiology tape application varies by indication, but the clinician typically follows these steps:

1. The area is cleaned of oils (if possible) and dried.

2. Excessive hair may be removed if it impedes application.

3. The middle 75% of the tape is stretched to an approximate tension (about 50%), then applied over the skin.

4. The ends are applied under no stretch.

5. The tape is rubbed to activate the adhesive.

6. Tape is reapplied every 3 to 7 days if its use is found to be beneficial.

   The utility of kinesiology tape is adjunct to manual techniques and rehabilitation with a physical therapist. Taping may be tried for a given set of patient symptoms and clinical findings because its use has no real adverse effect. Kinesiology tape is an adjunct that may benefit a subset of your patients.

Selected References

Farquharson C, Greig M. Kinesiology tape mediates soccer-simulated and local peroneal fatigue in soccer players. *Res Sports Med*. 2017;25(3):313-321.

Hashemirad F. Karimi N, Keshavarz R. The effect of Kinesio taping technique on trigger points of the piriformis muscle. *J Body Mov Ther*. 2016;20(4):807-814.

Kaplan S, Alpayci M, Karaman E, et al. Short-term effects of Kinesio taping in women with pregnancy-related low back pain: a randomized controlled clinical trial. *Med Sci Monit*. 2016;22:1297-1301.

Kelle B, Guzel R, Sakalli H. The effect of Kinesio taping application for acute non-specific low back pain: a randomized controlled clinical trial. *Clin Rehabil*. 2016;30(10):997-1003.

Kim MK, Shin YJ. Immediate effects of ankle balance taping with kinesiology tape for amateur soccer players with lateral ankle sprain: a randomized cross-over design. *Med Sci Monit*. 2017;23:5534-5541.

Köroğlu F, Çolak T, Polat MG. The effect of Kinesio® taping on pain, functionality, mobility and endurance in the treatment of chronic low back pain: a randomized controlled study. *J Back Musculoskelet Rehabil*. 2017;30(5):1087-1093.

Lim EC, Tay MG. Kinesio taping in musculoskeletal pain and disability that lasts for more than 4 weeks: is it time to peel off the tape and throw it out with the sweat? A systematic review with meta-analysis focused on pain and also methods of tape application. *Br J Sports Med*. 2015;49(24):1558-1566.

Myoung KK, Young Jun S. Immediate effects of ankle balance taping with kinesiology tape for amateur soccer players with lateral ankle sprain: a randomized cross-over design. *Med Sci Monit*. 2017;23:5534-5541.

Thelan MD, Dauber JA, Stoneman PD. The clinical efficacy of Kinesio tape for shoulder pain: a randomized, double-blinded, clinical trial. *J Orthop Sports Phys Ther*. 2008;38(7):389-395.

CHAPTER | 5

CODING AND BILLING FOR MANUAL MEDICINE

Documentation and coding for manual medicine interventions follows the very same conventions as any other procedure performed in the outpatient setting. A progress note must cover all the documentation requirements that support the indication for the procedure. The note MUST state the number of regions treated as well as the time spent "in constant attendance."

For billing, the diagnosis code used must be specific to the problem (for example, neck pain) but not to the level of muscle (such as scalene spasm). International Classification of Diseases, Tenth Revision, Clinical Modification (ICD-10-CM) codes should refer to the patient's symptoms or a definitive diagnosis, not a differential diagnosis. View manual medicine as a procedure; thus add the "modifier 25" code to your ICD-10 diagnosis code.

CPT Coding

One unique aspect of billing for manual medicine procedures is the CPT (Current Procedure Terminology) procedure code "97140 Manual Therapy Techniques (eg, mobilization/manipulation)." When you apply this CPT code, your electronic health record should ask for a quantity of *regions* treated. This is estimated based on the time to the halfway point of each interval, so if your visit is brief (approximately 15 minutes), bill for one unit; if the visit is more than 30 minutes, 2 units, and if more than 45 minutes, 3 units. Most commonly, for an initial visit, 2 units is a reasonable estimate.

CPT coding is time based and based on the *mid-point of the time period*. This may sound confusing, but using Table 5-1 or allowing just how long your visit is scheduled can help you choose the number of units.

TABLE 5.1 Time-Based CPT Coding

Minutes	Units	Reimbursement ($)
8-22	1	28.44
23-37	2	56.88
38-52	3	85.32

Documentation

Initial Visit

Documentation of the initial visit should include a chief complaint; full history of present illness; past medical, family, and social history (including new activities and work activity); and a review of systems that addresses your differential diagnosis. Your physical examination should include vital signs and musculoskeletal (range of motion [ROM], what might decrease/increase pain, spasm, deformities, etc), neurological, and other systems unique to your differential diagnosis. For example, if the patient has left neck pain, document the neck's ROM, palpation of the region (neck, clavicle, shoulder), AND a cardiac examination.

A procedure note should document your intervention, should speak to regions treated and method (stretch/relax or Muscle Energy Techniques, positional release, etc) used. Finally, include the length of time spent with the patient and document that you were present in "constant attendance."

Sample Procedure Note for Initial Visit

Informed Consent: After explaining the risks, benefits, and alternatives for the treatment, the patient gave verbal consent for the procedure.

Description of Procedure: While sitting, compression testing and Spurling test did not demonstrate radiculopathy. The patient was then placed in a supine position, resting comfortably. The cervical region was distracted, providing a decrease of symptoms. The anterior and posterior neck regions, along with the upper back, were all treated using MET/manual techniques. Trigger points in the trapezius were treated using positional release.

Outcomes/Complications: The patient noted 80% relief of the symptoms with no adverse effects; the patient continued to report pain relief after returning to a sitting position. Pain rated at a 7 before the procedure and was rated at a 3 afterward.

Instructions to Patient: The patient is instructed to use ice to the region for the next 24 hours if beneficial. The patient is given exercises to perform at home; they may begin ibuprofen 600 mg every 6 hours and is referred to physical therapy for further treatment.

Time: Total time spent in **constant attendance** with the patient performing manual therapy was 30 minutes.

Coding

99214 (based on complexity), Modifier 25, CPT: 97140 with units (2)

Follow-Up/Interval Visit

Should you see the patient again for an additional treatment, with no additional problems being discussed, you should minimally include an interval history on the course of the illness, what made symptoms better and worse, and physical examination noting range of motion, spasm, neurological deficits, etc. Another full procedure note should be documented (as earlier).

Coding

JUST 97140 with quantity (1, 2, 3); do not include an E & M code unless other problems are discussed.

Kinesiology Tape

Kinesiology tape can be billed but is not covered by all insurances. Documentation of kinesiology tape use should include justification (to support involved joint and healing, lymphatic drainage, etc). Describe the application technique (for example, an H-shaped application was applied to the upper back) and whether the patient felt decreased discomfort by the application.

   Coding

   CPT: Application code: 97799; supply code: 99070

   Each chapter will conclude with common diagnoses and suggested billing codes to assist in your completion of visit documentation.

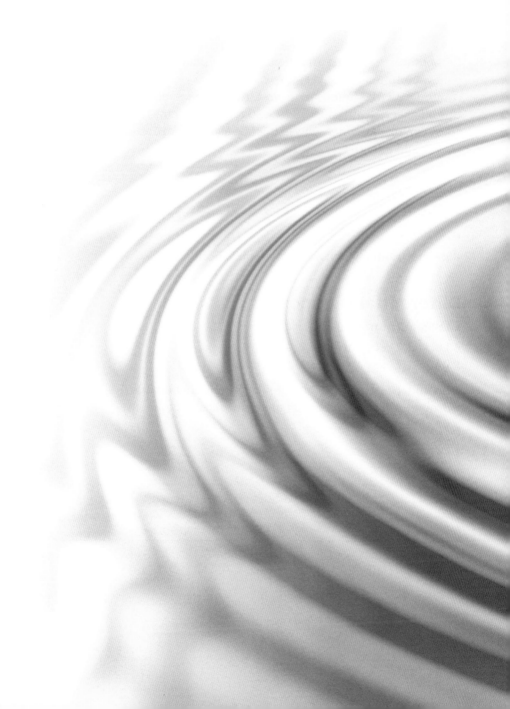

P A R T | 2
TREATMENTS

C H A P T E R | 6

NECK AND UPPER BACK PAIN

Computer screen time and the use of handheld phones has made upper back and neck pain a common finding. Acute pain can be related to a new activity (such as a new computer work station) or from a trauma such as a motor vehicle induced whiplash. Chronic neck strain can lead to secondary problems including headaches and decreased chest expansion which may influence asthma or mimic angina. Treating these regions is easy and effective.

History
- Work
- Activity
- Recent trauma (such as motor vehicle accident)

Differential Diagnosis
- Osteoarthritis of the cervical spine
- Locked facet joint
- Whiplash
- Shoulder/rotator cuff: subscapularis or supraspinatus dysfunction (impingement syndrome) can cause referred pain to the neck region
- Muscle spasm/torticollis
- Overuse

Alert: Left-sided symptoms need to be carefully evaluated for cardiac risk factors (including hypertension, hyperlipidemia, age older than 55 years, tobacco abuse, family history of early heart disease) and to rule out angina.

Physical Examination
Postural Assessment

- Assessment can be done in sitting or standing position.
- Determine the position of the head: neutral/forward/retracted and what position lessens symptoms.
- Try to get the patient back to neutral or normal posture.

Neck and Shoulder Range of Motion

- Have the patient move the neck to full flexion, extension, and side bending. Look for decreased range of motion (ROM).
- Have the patient move the both into forward flexion, extension, abduction. Look for muscle asymmetry and substitution to determine if the shoulder is the source of neck symptoms.
- If shoulder ROM is asymmetrical, perform more extensive shoulder assessment.
  - ⏵ Empty Can, Neer, Hawkins tests for impingement
  - ⏵ Apprehension testing for joint laxity

Palpation

- Palpate regions for muscle spasm and trigger points (Figure 6-1)
  - Trapezius

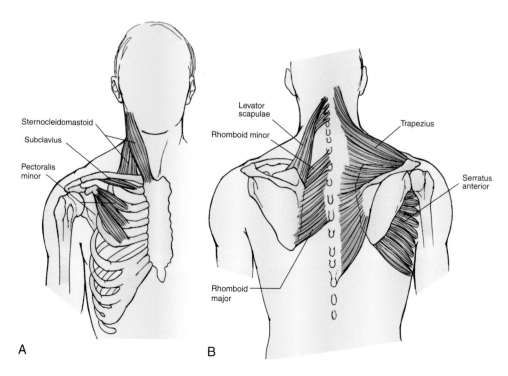

A   B

Figure 6-1 • Muscles of the neck and upper back. (Reprinted with permission from Oatis CA. *Kinesiology*. Baltimore: Wolters Kluwer; 2016.)

- Levator scapulae
- Sternocleidomastoid (SCM)
- Scalenes
- Temporomandibular Joint (TMJ) dysfunction
- Pectoralis minor

Special Tests
▶ Cervical Compression

Pain with compression may imply conditions such as herniated nucleus pulposus, facet arthropathy, and degenerative joint disease/osteoarthritis.

- Have patient in neutral. Place your interlocked fingers over the head.
- Use your body weight to gently push down, asking the patient if this action reproduces their symptoms, implying referred pain to the affected upper trapezius and arm.

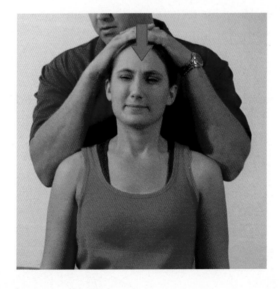

Spurling Test

- With the patient sitting, rotate the head toward the affected side and mildly side bend it toward the same side, then provide downward compression.
- If this maneuver reproduces symptoms, nerve impingement is likely.

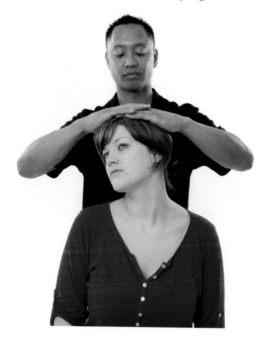

⊙ Cervical Distraction

Sitting

- Place your hands on each side of the neck with your index fingers under the mandible and lift up.
- A decrease in symptoms implies nerve impingement from HNP.

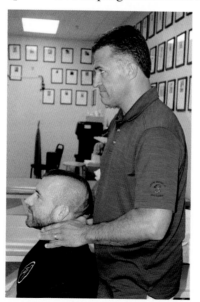

Supine

- Place your hands under the occiput and on the forehead and pull caudally.
- A decrease in symptoms implies nerve impingement from HNP.

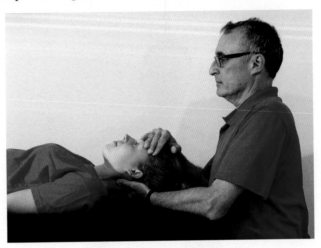

Treatments

> **Remember the Rules**
> 1. Move to a position of less pain
> 2. Stretch the SHORTENED muscle
> 3. Treat the region (above and below pain)
> 4. Tape to support neutral position
> 5. Support definitive treatment (physical therapy, orthopedics, neurosurgery)

Postural Correction

- Gently move the patient to neutral and relax.
- Then have the patient attempt to correct posture on his or her own.

Mobilization

▶ Stretching Strap or Towel

- The goal is to find the level that enables more motion with less pain.
- Place a towel or strap over the point of maximal tenderness and move through ROM, then above and below that point.

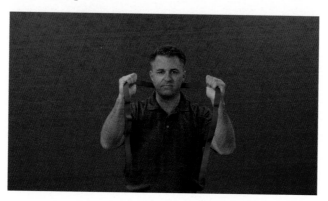

- Apply anterior pressure with the strap or towel.
- Moving your hands in coordination with the head, move the head through ROM: flexion (forward) and extension (backward) and side bending for 10 repetitions.

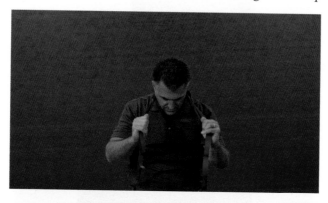

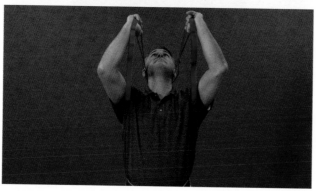

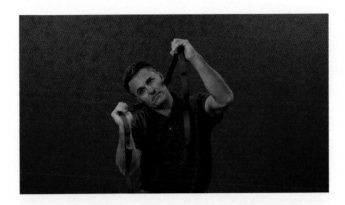

Chin Tuck

- Place a rolled towel under the chin and gently press the jaw down into the towel. Relax and repeat.
- Reposition head and towel slightly to find best pain-relieving position.

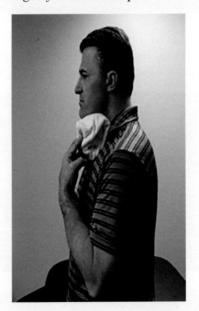

Manual Therapy

▶ Anterior Neck and Upper Back

- With the patient supine, have the patient put the uninvolved hand on their sternum and place your hand on top of the patient's hand.
- Place your other hand on the side of the patient's head.
- Rotate the head away from affected side to end point (furthest motion before causing pain, muscle guarding, or spasm).
- Hold the head and sternum while the patient attempts to turn their head back to the midline with 10% effort for three belly breaths.

- As the patient relaxes, turn the head further away from the side of discomfort by taking up the slack; then repeat for a total of three cycles.

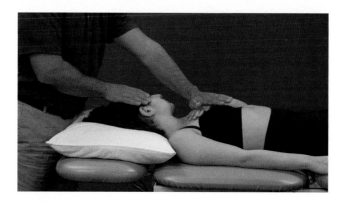

▶ Lateral Neck and Trapezius

- Have the patient side bend the neck away from the involved side and move the involved shoulder inferiorly.
- With one hand, hold the head in place. Cross your arms and with your other hand, hold the shoulder down.

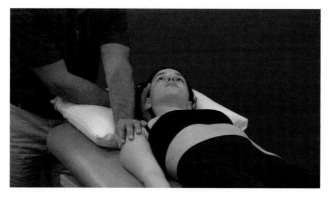

- Ask the patient to move the ear toward the shoulder with 10% effort against resistance while taking three belly breaths, then relax.
- Move the head and shoulder further apart. Repeat for total of three cycles.

▶ Levator Scapulae

- With the patient standing, move the involved arm posteriorly and medially.
- Ask the patient to side flex the neck away from the involved side, rotate away from the affected side, and forward flex the neck to the end point (like trying to "look at your hip").
- Ask the patient to hold their head in place with the uninvolved hand.
- Place your hand on the involved shoulder to stabilize.

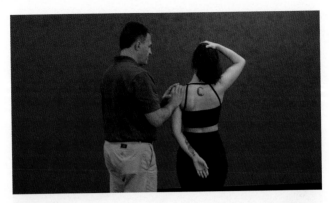

- Have the patient try to bring the ear toward the involved shoulder with 10% effort while taking three belly breaths. Then relax.
- Take up the slack in the neck and repeat these steps for a total of three cycles.

▶ Medial Upper Back: Rhomboids

- Have the patient lie on the unaffected side with the hips and knees bent 90 degrees.
- Place your arm under the axilla.
- Reach across and grasp the medial border of the scapula with both hands.

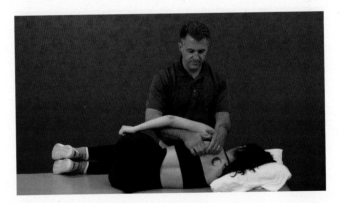

- Gently rotate the scapula toward you, remembering the scapula rotates with its inferior aspect moving more laterally than its superior aspect.
- Ask the patient to use 10% effort to move the shoulder back toward midline ("pinch your shoulders together") into your hand while taking three belly breaths, then relax.

- Move the scapula further laterally.

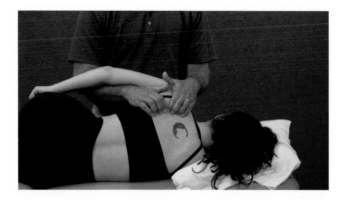

- Repeat these steps for a total of three stretch-relax cycles.

▶ Upper Back/Trunk Rotators

- Have the patient sit up tall on the edge of the table and rotate the upper body away from the involved side.
- Place one hand on the posterior aspect of the involved shoulder, the other on the anterior aspect of the uninvolved shoulder.

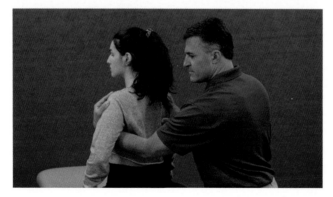

- Ask the patient to rotate back against your hand on the involved side, using 10% effort while taking three belly breaths.

- Have the patient relax and sit tall while you further rotate their spine away from the involved side.

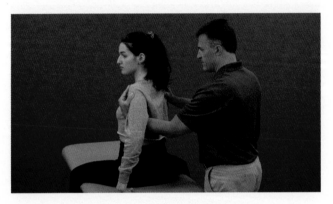

- Repeat these steps for a total of three stretch-relax cycles.

▶ Upper and Mid Back (Quadratus Lumborum)

- With the patient sitting, place the uninvolved elbow on their thigh or on a pillow over the thigh and the involved hand on the side of the head and lean away from the involved side.

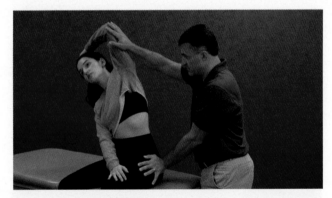

- Help the patient lean toward their limit and while holding the patient's hip and elbow at the limit, ask the patient to use 10% effort to push against your hand with their elbow while taking three belly breaths, then relaxing.

- As the patient relaxes, move the patient further into the stretch away from the involved side.

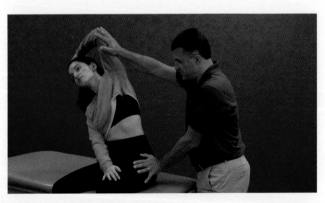

- Repeat these steps for a total of three stretch-relax cycles.

▶ Strain/Counterstain

- This technique is performed if trigger points are present.
- Have the patient lie supine while you palpate the trapezius to identify trigger points and gently compress.

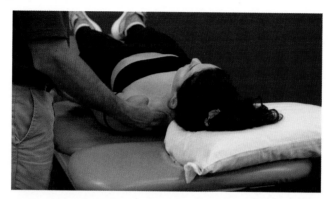

- Side bend the head toward the involved side to further relax the trapezius.
- Move the patient's arm in all directions until the trigger point completely softens.

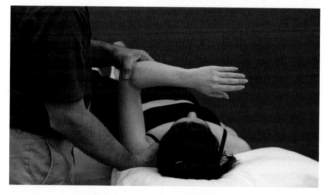

- Hold this position for up to 90 seconds while the patient takes slow belly breaths and you feel for the trigger point releasing.
- After 90 seconds, the clinician should move the patient's arm back to their side.

Kinesiology Taping

▶ Neck Support

- Measure three 10-inch strips of tape.
- *For the first piece of tape:* Place the first 2 inches at the level of the inferior aspect of the scapula just lateral to the spine.
- Using 25% to 50% stretch, apply the tape vertically.
- Apply the last 2 inches without tension.

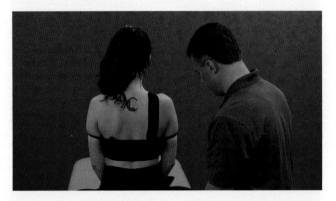

- *For the second piece of tape:* Repeat on the opposite side of the spine.
- *For the third piece of tape:* Place the first 2 inches of the tape horizontally on the medial aspect of the trapezius without any tension.
- Using a 25% to 50% stretch, apply the tape across the midline to the opposite trapezius.
- Apply the last 2 inches without any tension.
- Rub the tape to activate it.

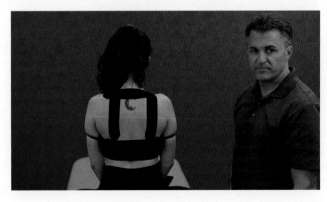

▶ Postural Support

- Measure 2 strips, one from the top of one shoulder to below the scapula on the opposite side.

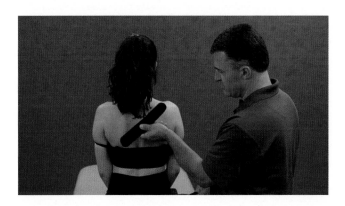

- *For the first piece of tape:* Place the first 2 inches on the trapezius without any tension.
- Using 25% to 50% stretch, apply the middle section across the spine to below the opposite scapula.
- Apply the last 2 inches of the tape without any stretch.

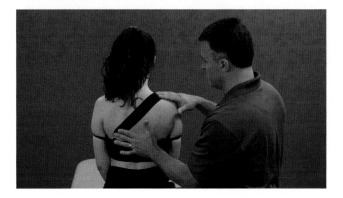

- *For the second piece of tape:* Repeat on the opposite side and then rub to activate the adhesive.

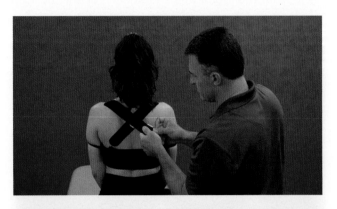

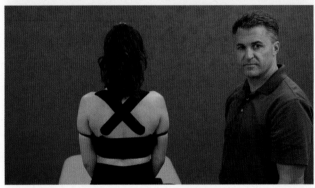

▶ Upper Back Support

- Measure three 8-inch strips of tape.
- *For the first piece of tape:* Place the first 2 inches vertically at the level of the inferior aspect of the scapula, just lateral to the spine.
- Using 25% to 50% stretch, apply the tape vertically.
- Apply the last 2 inches without tension.
- *For the second piece of tape:* Repeat the tape application on the other side of the spine.

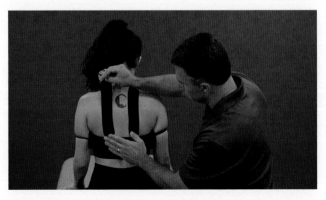

- *For the third piece of tape:* At the level of patient's discomfort, place the first 2 inches horizontally at the scapula's medial edge without tension.
- Using 25% to 50% stretch, apply the tape horizontally.
- Apply the last 2 inches without tension.

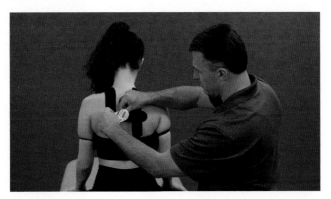

- Rub to activate the adhesive.

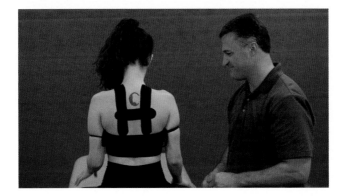

Treatment Summary

Mobilization

Stretching Strap or Towel

1.
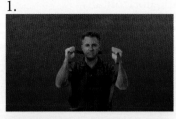

2.
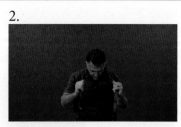

3.
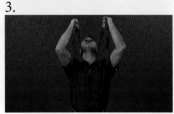

4.
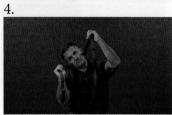

Manual Therapy

Anterior Neck and Upper Back

1.
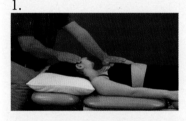

Lateral Neck and Trapezius

1.
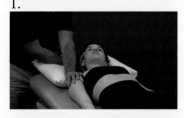

Levator Scapulae

1.
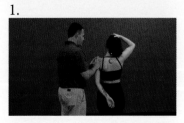

Medial Upper Back: Rhomboids

1.

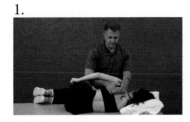

2.

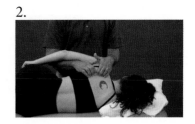

Upper Back/ Trunk Rotators

1.

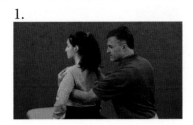

2.

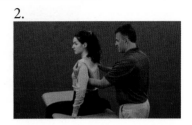

Upper and Mid Back

1.

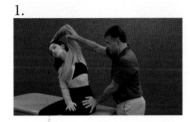

2.

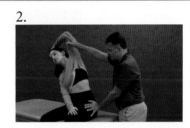

Strain/ Counterstain

1.

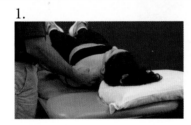

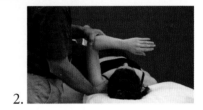

2.

Kinesiology Taping

Neck Support

1.

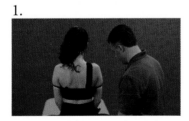

2.

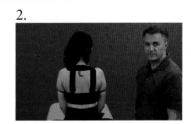

Postural Support

1.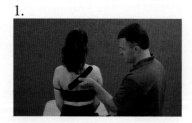

2.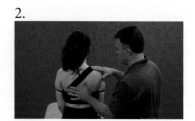

3.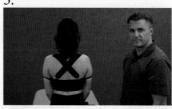

Upper Back Support

1.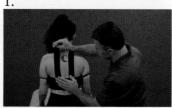

2.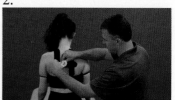

3.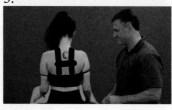

Sample Procedure Notes and Coding

Procedure:	**E/M**: 99213 or 99214 **ICD** 10: M54.2 Cervicalgia & Modifier 25 **CPT**: 97140 – Manual therapy techniques 1 or more regions	
	Minutes	**Units Reported**
	8-22	1
	23-37	2
	38-52	3
	53-67	4
	--99070 – Supplies and Materials: applied by health care professional (list supplies/materials used)	
Informed consent	After explaining the risks, benefits, and alternatives for the treatment, the patient gave verbal consent for the procedure	
Description of Procedure		
Outcomes/ Complications	The patient's symptoms reduced by ____% and there were no complications	
Instructions to Patient	Use neck and upper back exercise sheet and schedule evaluation with Physical Therapy	
Time	Total time spent in **constant attendance** with the patient performing manual therapies: ____ minutes	

Mobilization: Stretching Strap or Towel

- Place a towel or strap over the most painful area.
- Using both hands, pull strap or towel forward to apply pressure to the painful area.
- Moving your hands in coordination with the head, gently move the head forward, backward, and side to side for 10 repetitions.

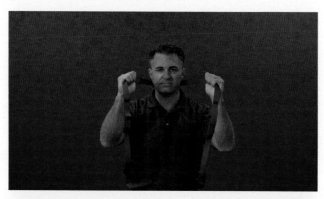

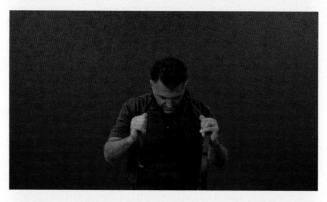

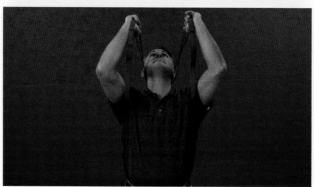

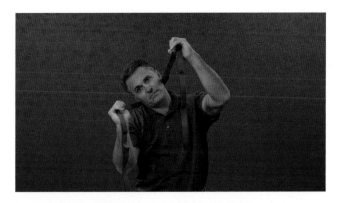

Chin Tuck

- Place a rolled towel under the chin and gently press the jaw down into the towel. Relax and repeat.
- Reposition the head and towel slightly to find the best pain-relieving position.

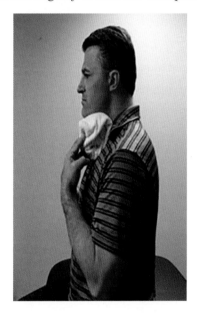

Mobilization: Tennis or Softball

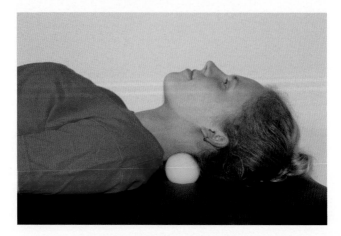

- Rest area of tenderness on tennis ball, applying amount of pressure that produces muscle relaxation; this should be relaxing, not painful.

Scalenes Stretch

- Grasp side of chair on affected side.
- Turn your head to look in the opposite armpit and take three belly breaths.

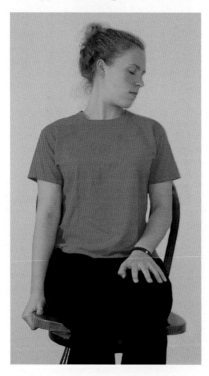

- Next, gently let the ear on the uninvolved side move toward your shoulder for three belly breaths.

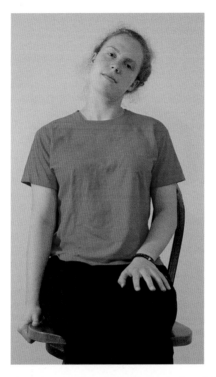

- Finally, turn your head and look up over the affected shoulder and take three belly breaths.

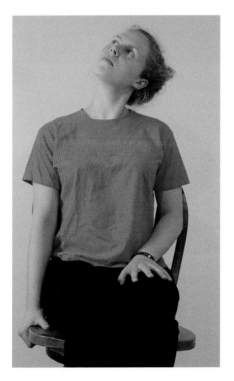

Wall Stretch

- Stand against a wall.
- Pull the shoulder blades together and hold for 5 seconds, relax, and repeat five times.

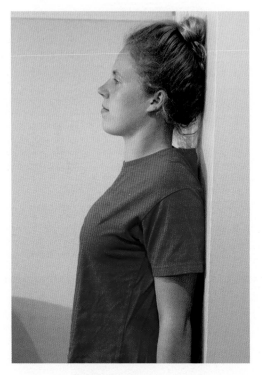

Upper Trapezius Ball Self Massage

- Place two tennis balls in a sock and tie a knot in the end.
- Place this sock between the neck and shoulder area and use body pressure to push up, down or side-to-side to massage tight areas. Some pain is okay.

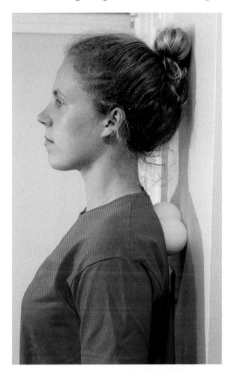

Doorway Stretch

- Stand in a corner or a doorway with your arms positioned as shown in the image.
- Move one foot forward (to avoid putting all weight through the shoulders).
- Slowly lean forward until a stretch is felt across your chest.
- Make sure to maintain good posture throughout the stretch, with the shoulders back, the head up, and the abdominal muscles tight.
- Hold for 5 seconds.
- Relax and repeat these steps five times.

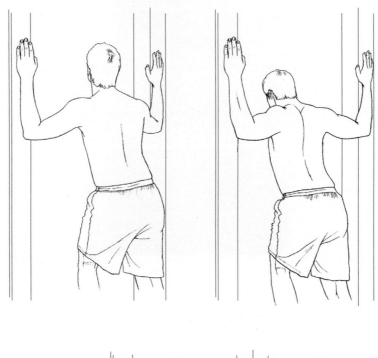

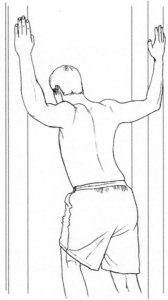

Floor Stretch

- Lie down on a vertical foam roller.
- Tighten your abdominal muscles to keep the back from arching up; pinch your shoulders.
- Make sure your palms are facing up.
- Keeping your arms relatively straight, slide your arms along the floor up and down until a stretch is felt across the chest.
- Hold the tight areas for 5 seconds. Repeat five times.

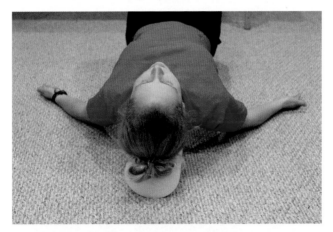

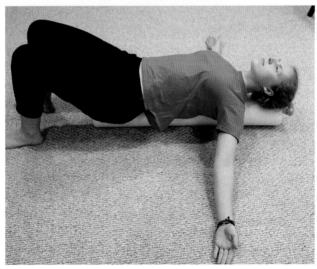

Mid Back: Stretch With Dowel

- While standing, hold a stick behind your back with your elbows (as shown).
- Slowly turn your upper body to each side while keeping your hips facing forward. You should feel a stretch through your midback.
- Throughout the motion, keep your spine straight, head up, shoulders back, and abdominals tight.
- Repeat these steps for five full rotations.

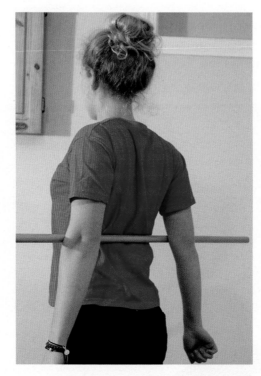

Levator Scapulae Self Stretch

- Sit on a table or chair that allows you to grab behind (as shown) with the involved arm.
- Using the other arm, reach over and grab the side of your head and gently pull your ear towards your shoulder till you feel a gentle stretch.
- Hold this position and take three deep breaths, then relax and repeat three times.

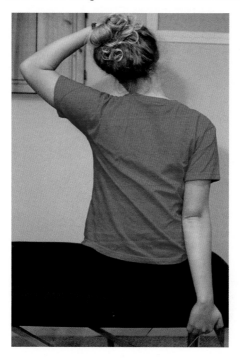

Door-Frame Stretch

- Grasp a door frame or wall at eye level, as shown.

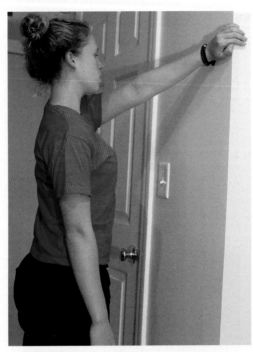

- Rotate the uninvolved shoulder toward the wall and gently lean in; take three belly breaths, then relax.
- Move your arm down to shoulder level and repeat, then down to stomach level, and repeat three times.

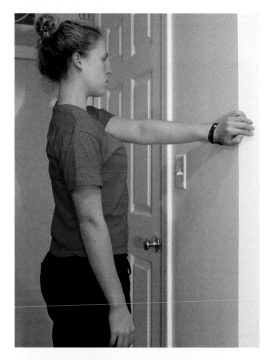

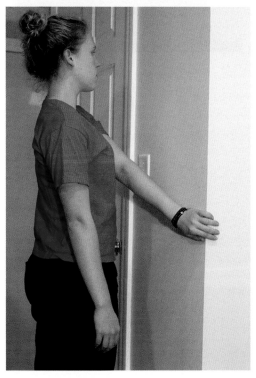

Rhomboid and Middle Trapezius Self Stretch

- With the arm and elbow flexed 90 degrees, move the arm toward midline until limit is reached.
- Grasp your elbow with your other hand, then push your elbow against the hand, holding resistance for five counts. Then relax, pull the elbow further in front of you, and repeat five times.

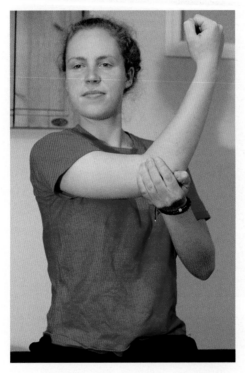

Selected References

Areeuodomwong P, Wongrat W, Neammesri N, Thongsakul T. A randomized controlled trial on the long-term effects of proprioceptive neuromuscular facilitation training, on pain-related outcomes and back muscle activity, in patients with chronic low back pain. *Musculoskeletal Care*. 2017;15(3):218-229.

Burns DK, Wells MR. Gross range of motion in the cervical spine: the effects of osteopathic muscle energy technique in asymptomatic subjects. *J Am Osteopath Assoc*. 2006;106(3):137-142.

Côté P, Wong JJ, Sutton D, et al. Management of neck pain and associated disorders: a clinical practice guideline from the Ontario Protocol for Traffic Injury Management (OPTIMa) Collaboration *Eur Spine J*. 2016;25(7):2000-2022.

Espí-López GV, Arnal-Gómez A, Arbós-Berenguer T, et al. Effectiveness of physical therapy in patients with tension-type headache: literature review. *J Jpn Phys Ther Assoc*. 2014;17(1):31-38.

Wong CK, Abraham T, Karimi P, et al. Strain counterstrain technique to decrease tender point palpation pain compared to control conditions: a systematic review with meta-analysis. *J Bodyw Mov Ther*. 2014;18(2):165.

Wong JJ, Shearer HM, Mior S, et al. Are manual therapies, passive physical modalities, or acupuncture effective for the management of patients with whiplash-associated disorders or neck pain and associated disorders? An update of the bone and joint decade task force on neck pain and its associated disorders by the OPTIMa collaboration. *Spine J*. 2016;16(12):1598-1630.

Figure Credits

Spurling Test figure reprinted with permission from Bucci C. Condition-Specific Massage Therapy. Philadelphia: Wolters Kluwer; 2011 with permission.

Doorway stretch figures reprinted from Anatomical Chart Company with permission from Wolters Kluwer.

C H A P T E R | 7
SHOULDER

Introduction

In most adults who present with atraumatic shoulder pain, symptoms arise from impingement syndromes (previously called rotator cuff tendonitis). These symptoms become more common as patients age.

The rotator cuff is made up of four muscle-tendon structures (supraspinatus, infraspinatus, teres minor, subscapularis) (Figure 7-1). Their combined activity is to move the shoulder through space and maintain the joint's integrity. The symptoms of impingement can be managed initially by manual techniques. When followed by an aggressive physical therapy program, impingment syndrome can often be cured without surgery. Trauma-related shoulder pain is also often effectively treated without surgery, but an accurate diagnosis is needed as well as the recognition that failure to resolve may result in operative correction.

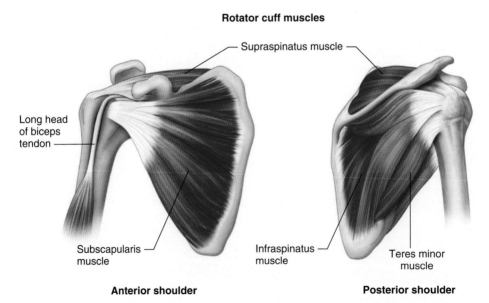

Figure 7-1 • Rotator cuff anatomy. (Reprinted from Beggs I. *Musculoskeletal Ultrasound*. Philadelphia: Wolters Kluwer; 2013 with permission.)

Diagnosis

Differential Diagnosis

- Impingement (rotator cuff tendonitis)
- Derangement/labral tear
- Infection
- Angina (left shoulder)
- Rhomboid spasm

History Consistent With Impingement Syndrome (Rotator Cuff Tendonitis)

- Onset without history of trauma.
- Pain initially bothersome with abduction movements; progresses to painful with reaching over head and may cause awakening while sleeping.

Alert: If left arm symptoms are present, rule out anginal equivalent/cardiovascular etiology

Testing for Impingement Syndrome (Rotator Cuff Tendonitis)

Range of Motion: Active and Passive

- Ask the patient to keep elbows straight and abduct the arms to horizontal and ultimately over their heads, looking for asymmetry of muscle use.
- If there is a significant asymmetry have the patient relax and move that extremity through passive range of motion through abduction.

▶ Empty Can

- Pronate the patient's arms, moving the arms off center to 45 degrees with the thumbs down.
- Place your hands on the patient's wrists and resist the patient's attempt to raise their arms, comparing sides for weakness of involved side and/or if the maneuver causes pain.

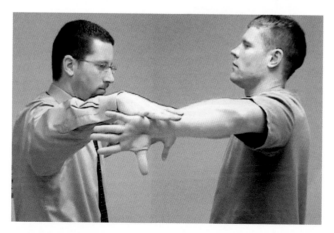

▶ Neer Test

- Move the arm in forward flexion, first through active and then passive flexion, noting if and when the patient has pain.
- If pain occurs with active range on motion (ROM) only, consider impingement. If pain occurs with both active and passive ROM, consider adhesive capsulitis.

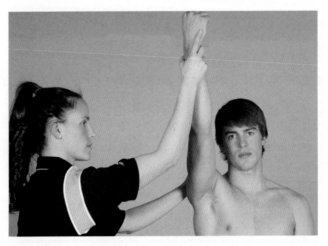

▶ Hawkins Test

- Forward flex the patient's shoulder and bend the elbow to 90 degrees. Support the patient's elbow and wrist with your hands.
- Rotate the patient's forearm to 90 degrees, then beyond the horizontal, looking to determine if moving past horizontal induces pain or discomfort. If pain or discomfort occur, impingement is likely the cause.

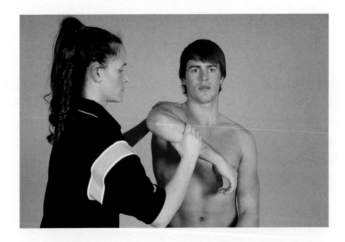

Testing for Joint Laxity/Subluxation/Dislocation

▶ Apprehension Testing

- With the patient sitting or supine, abduct the patient's arm to 90 degrees and bend the elbow.
- GENTLY move the patient's hand posteriorly, then ask the patient to press forward against resistance.
- Then, have them press posteriorly against resistance.
- If either movement makes the patient feel uncomfortable or agitated, consider a lax joint.

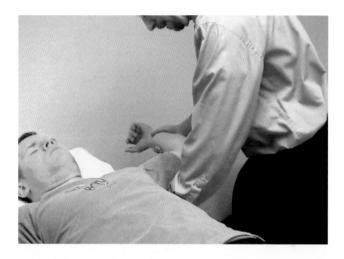

Remember the Rules

1. Move to a position of less pain and apply trigger point care
2. Stretch the SHORTENED muscle
3. Treat the region (above and below pain)
4. Tape to support neutral position
5. Support definitive treatment (physical therapy, orthopedics, neurosurgery)

Treatment
Mobilization

▶ **Pain/Restriction with Abduction: Supraspinatus Treatment**

- While supine, have the patient forward flex the affected arm to their limit. The patient's thumb should be pointing behind the patient's head.
- Hold resistance against the patient's wrist and shoulder.

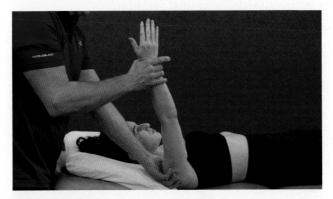

- Have the patient, using 10% effort, try to move the arm back to their side, taking three belly breaths and then relaxing.
- Move the patient's arm further back.

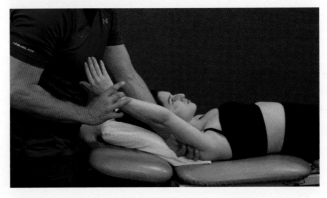

- Repeat these steps for a total of three stretch-relax cycles.
- Move the arm back to the patient's side.
- Abduct the arm with the elbow extended until the patient has pain or reaches a limit.

- Grasp the arm at the wrist and elbow and ask the patient to push with 10% effort against resistance while taking three belly breaths, then relax.

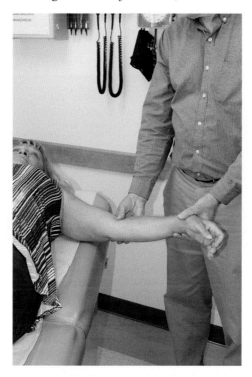

- Move the arm into further abduction.
- Repeat for a total of three stretch/relax cycles.

▶ Pain/Restriction With External Rotation: Subscapularis Treatment

- With the patient supine, flex their arm to 30 degrees, abduct the shoulder to 30 degrees, keeping the flexed elbow anterior to the ribs.

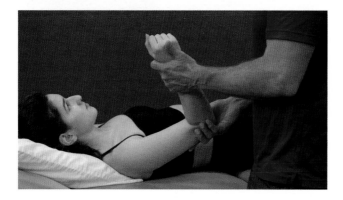

- Support the elbow with one hand and grasp the wrist with the other; then rotate the forearm into supination.
- Externally rotate the shoulder, including the humerus, posteriorly until it reaches an end point. (The shoulder should rotate. Do not apply leverage or torque to the medial elbow.)

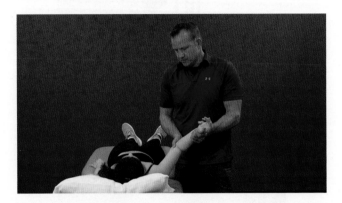

- While holding their wrist and elbow, ask the patient to use 10% effort to internally rotate the shoulder by pushing into your hands.
- Ask the patient to take three belly breaths and then relax.
- Continue to rotate the shoulder posteriorly and repeat for three stretch-relax cycles.

▶ Pain/Restriction With Internal Rotation: Infraspinatus and Teres Minor

- Position the patient prone with the shoulder supported by a pillow or a rolled towel and with the arm bent and hanging off the table.

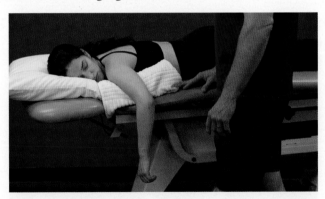

- Keep the upper arm at 90 degrees while rotating the palm up toward the ceiling until the end point.

- Ask the patient to push the back of their wrist toward the floor, using 10% effort, against resistance while taking three belly breaths and then relaxing.

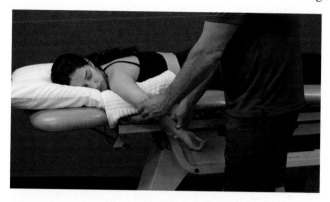

- As the patient relaxes, move the arm further into rotation toward the ceiling.
- Repeat these steps for a total of three stretch-relax cycles.

▶ Lateral Neck and Trapezius

- Have the patient side bend the neck away from involved side and move the involved shoulder inferiorly.
- With one hand, hold the head in place. Cross your arms and with your other hand, hold the shoulder down.
- Ask the patient to move the ear toward the shoulder with 10% effort against resistance while taking three belly breaths, then relax.

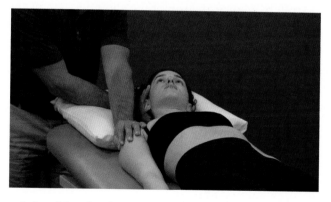

- Move the head and shoulder further apart. Repeat for total of three cycles.

▶ Kinesiology Taping for Shoulder Pain

- Measure two strips of tape from the anterior aspect of the humeral head to 2 inches beyond the medial aspect of the lower scapula.
- Have the patient gently squeeze the scapulae together.
- Place 2 inches of the first piece of tape over the anterior humeral head without tension.
- Then apply 25% to 50% tension and pull the tape around the lateral aspect of shoulder and across to just beyond the medial aspect of the lower scapula.

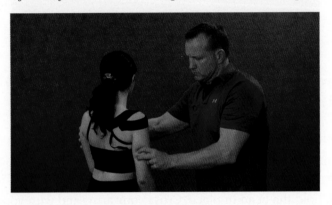

- Apply the last 2 inches of tape without any tension.
- With the second piece of tape, apply 2 inches anteriorly just medial to the end of the first piece of tape.
- Using 25% to 50% stretch, go over the top of the shoulder, and at the top of the scapula, move the tape medially and down the medial aspect of the scapula.
- Apply the last 2 inch of tape without tension.
- Rub the tape to activate the adhesive.

Sample Procedure Notes and Coding

Procedure:	**E/M:** 99213 or 99214 **ICD 10:** M75.40 Impingement syndrome of unspecified shoulder M75.00 Adhesive capsulitis of unspecified shoulder **CPT:** 97140—Manual therapy techniques one or more regions
	<table><tr><th>Minutes</th><th>Units Reported</th></tr><tr><td>8-22</td><td>1</td></tr><tr><td>23-37</td><td>2</td></tr><tr><td>38-52</td><td>3</td></tr><tr><td>53-67</td><td>4</td></tr></table>
	99070—Supplies and Materials: applied by health care professional (list supplies/materials used)
Informed consent	After explaining the risks, benefits and alternatives for the treatment, the patient gave verbal consent for the procedure.
Description of Procedure	
Outcomes/ Complications	The patient's symptoms reduced by ___% and there were no complications.
Instructions to Patient	
Time	Total time spent in **constant attendance** with the patient performing manual therapies: XX minutes

Mobilization With Softball

- Place a softball over the tender spots.
- Move your arm forward in flexion and then back to your side.
- Repeat this range of motion five times.

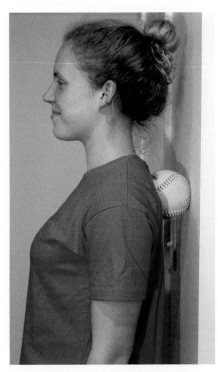

Shoulder Range of Motion

- Stand up straight, keep your head still, and squeeze your shoulder blades together.
- Hold this position for 5 seconds.
- Repeat these steps 10 times.

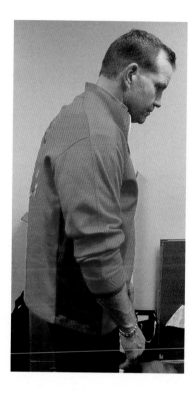 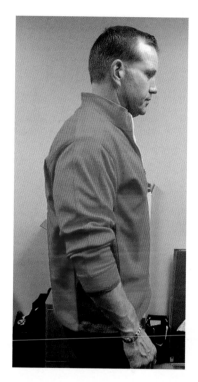

Rows (Isometric Scapular Engagement)

- Stand up straight and keep your head centered over your shoulders.
- Bend your elbows forward.
- Pull your elbows back and squeeze your shoulder blades together.
- Hold this position for 5 seconds.
- Repeat these steps 10 times.

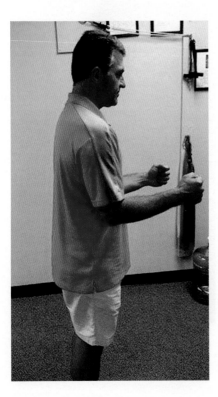 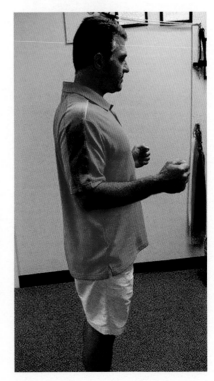

Self-Stretch

- Sit with your elbow bent and supported on a table.
- Using your other hand, rotate the arm to the side until the muscles get tight, keeping your spine straight.
- Take three belly breaths, relax, and repeat these steps 10 times.

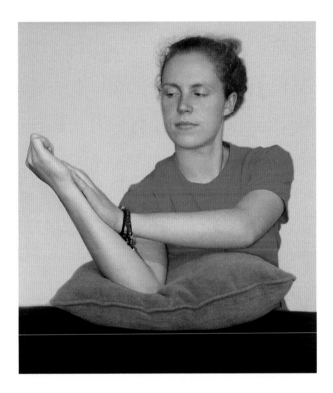

Bilateral Doorway (Pectoralis/Anterior Capsule) Stretch

- Stand in a corner or a doorway with your arms positioned as shown in the image.
- Move one foot forward (to avoid putting all weight through the shoulders).
- Slowly lean forward until a stretch is felt across your chest.
- Make sure to maintain good posture throughout the stretch, with the shoulders back, the head up, and the abdominal muscles tight.
- Hold for 5 seconds.
- Relax and repeat these steps five times.

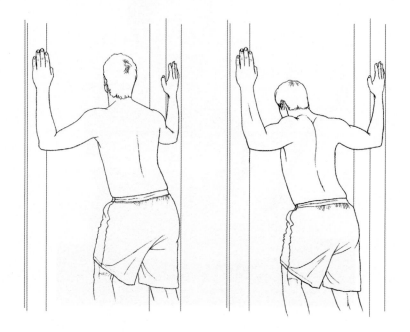

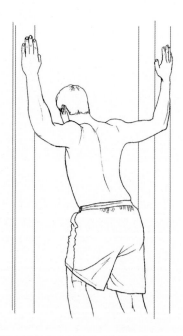

Door-Frame Stretch

- Grasp a door frame or wall edge at eye level with the painful arm, as shown.
- Rotate the uninvolved shoulder toward the wall and gently lean in; take three belly breaths, then relax.
- Move your arm down to shoulder level and repeat, then down to stomach level, and repeat three times.

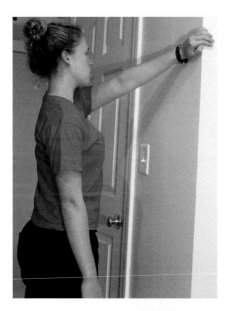
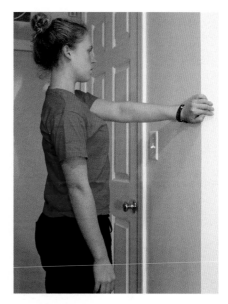

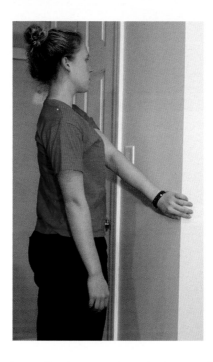

Subscapularis Stretch With Dowel

- Move your painful arm out to the side and bend the elbow.
- Grab the dowel with your upper hand, holding the stick behind your elbow.
- Grab the bottom of the dowel with your other hand, and pull the stick to move the upper hand backward.
- Take three belly breaths, relax, and then repeat these steps 10 times.

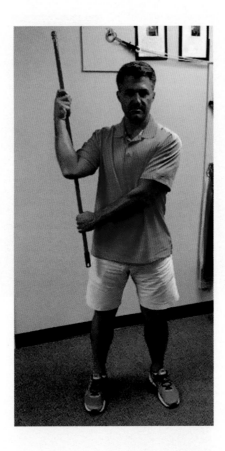

Subscapularis Stretching Strap

- Hold the strap in front of you with the pain-free hand and place the strap over the pain-free shoulder, letting the strap hang behind your back.
- Place your painful arm behind your back and grasp the strap.

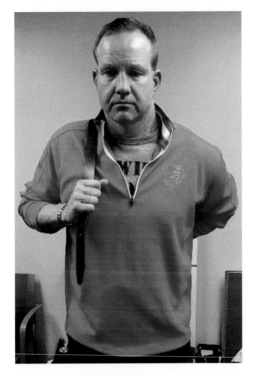

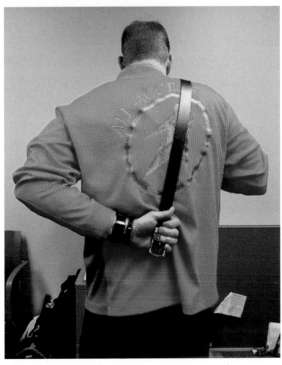

- Stand up straight; with your good arm, pull the strap down in front which will pull the painful arm toward the middle and your hand up, stretching your shoulder.

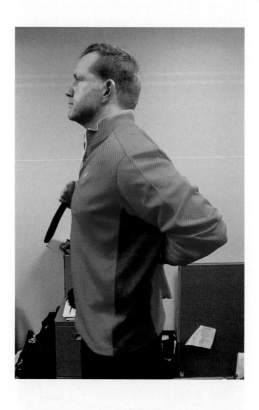

Rhomboid and Middle Trapezius Self-Stretch

- With the painful arm and elbow flexed 90 degrees, move the arm toward midline until limit is reached.
- Grasp your elbow with your other hand, then push your elbow against the hand, holding resistance for 5 counts. Then relax and repeat five times.

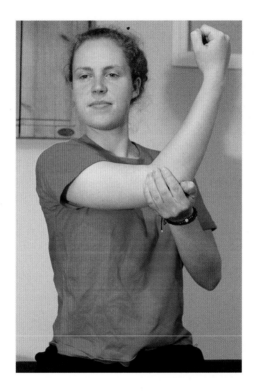

Selected References

Laudner KG, Wenig M, Selkow NM, Williams J, Post E. Forward shoulder posture in collegiate swimmers: a comparative analysis of muscle-energy techniques. *Athl Train*. 2015;50(11):1133-1139.

Moore SD, Laudner KG, McLoda TA, Shaffer MA. The immediate effects of muscle energy technique on posterior shoulder tightness: a randomized controlled trial. *J Orthop Sports Phys Ther*. 2011;41(6):400-407.

Reed ML, Begaller RL, Laudner KG. Acute effects of muscle energy technique and joint mobilization on shoulder tightness in youth throwing athletes: a randomized controlled trial. *Int J Sports Phys Ther*. 2018;13(6):1024-1031.

Figure Credits

Neer test images reprinted from Anderson MK. Foundations of Athletic Training. 6th ed. Baltimore: Wolters Kluwer; 2016 with permission.

Hawkins test images reprinted from Anderson MK. Foundations of Athletic Training. 6th ed. Baltimore: Wolters Kluwer; 2016 with permission.

CHAPTER | 8
ACUTE CHEST DISCOMFORT

Introduction

Anytime a patient hints at "chest pain," we focus on the heart first, then maybe the lungs. Yet in adults, musculoskeletal causes of chest pain are very common and are often related to activities such as computer work or lifting. New parents are prone to costochondritis from lifting a rapidly growing baby from a crib. Sitting with an ill-situated computer or at any workstation can induce what is called "upper crossed syndrome."

Be aware of risk factors for cardiovascular disease or pulmonary emboli. When these conditions are ruled out, focus on other syndromes, including upper crossed syndrome, first rib syndrome, and costochondritis.

Differential Diagnosis

• Angina (left side)

> **Alert:** Left-sided symptoms need to be carefully evaluated for cardiac risk factors (including hypertension, hyperlipidemia, age older than 55 years, tobacco abuse, family history of early heart disease) and to rule out angina.

• Pulmonary embolism

> **Alert:** Chest pain associated with shortness of breath, tachycardia, hemoptysis, and recent long immobilization (such as a car or plane ride, cast, surgery, history of being bedridden) requires full evaluation to rule out pulmonary embolism.

• Upper Crossed Syndrome
  • Tight trapezius and levator scapula in the upper back with tight pectoral muscles of the chest, leading to head shifting forward and chest shifting backward
  • Results in rounded shoulders; may cause posterior pelvic tilt (Figure 8-1)
  • Seen in those who work long hours in front of a computer screen and in women with pendulous breasts
  • Symptoms include headache, shoulder and neck pain, anterior chest pain, lower back pain and achiness with driving long distances

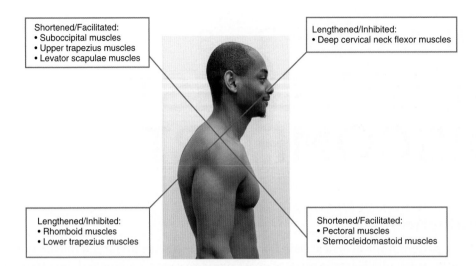

Shortened/Facilitated:
• Suboccipital muscles
• Upper trapezius muscles
• Levator scapulae muscles

Lengthened/Inhibited:
• Deep cervical neck flexor muscles

Lengthened/Inhibited:
• Rhomboid muscles
• Lower trapezius muscles

Shortened/Facilitated:
• Pectoral muscles
• Sternocleidomastoid muscles

Figure 8-1 • Upper crossed syndrome. (Reprinted from Donnelly JM, et al. *Travell, Simons & Simons' Myofascial Pain and Dysfunction*. Baltimore: Wolters Kluwer; 2018 with permission.)

- Palpate for overactive and tender points on the trapezius, levator scapulae and pectoralis major and minor, rhomboids, steroncleidomastoids, and pectoralis muscles
- Lengthened and tender muscles in upper crossed syndrome include the rhomboids, lower trapezius and neck flexors. Shortened muscles include the upper trapezius, levator scapulae, and sterocleidomastoids and pectoralis muscles.
- Costochondritis
  - Signs and symptoms include anterior chest wall pain and tenderness of the costochondral and sternoclavicular regions, most often affecting the second to the fifth costal cartilages.
  - Palpate costochondral junctions; pain is usually sharp, achy, or pressure-like, involving multiple (and mostly unilateral second to fifth) costal cartilages.
  - Pain can be exacerbated by upper body movements and exertional activities.
- First Rib Syndrome and Dysfunction
  - May be due to muscular dysfunction or a true subluxation (rib move out of joint)
  - Can be a cause of neck, shoulder, arm, and back pain
  - Etiology
    - Results from tight muscles in the neck from overuse or posture (especially in those using cell phones or pads)
    - May also be related to those using only the chest muscles to breathe, rather than chest and abdominals
  - Often associated with upper crossed syndrome (tight levator scapulae, trapezius, and pectoralis muscles)
  - Related to thoracic outlet syndrome: a constellation of symptoms that affect the head, neck, shoulders, and upper extremities caused by compression of the neurovascular structures (brachial plexus and subclavian vessels) at the thoracic outlet, specifically in the area superior to the first rib and posterior to the clavicle.

Symptoms and History

- Discomfort with raising arm overhead/combing hair
- Pain or difficulty turning your head side to side
- Hand/arm paresthesia
- Unsuccessful shoulder pain treatment
- More common in stomach sleepers (often with arm under pillow), in racket sport players, weight lifters

Physical Examination

- Rule out thoracic outlet syndrome—test for weakness of the muscles of the hand, especially the thumb.
- Adson sign: radial pulse in the arm is lost throughout abduction and external rotation of the shoulder (due to subclavian artery compression).
- Palpate the area behind the medial clavicle on the affected side for tenderness and asymmetry compared with the other side.
- Palpate the levator scapulae, trapezius, and insertions of pectoralis minor for tenderness.

Treatment

Remember the Rules

- Move the patient to a position of less pain and apply trigger point care.
- Stretch the *shortened* muscle.
- Treat the region (above and below pain).
- Tape to support a neutral position.
- Support definitive treatment (physical therapy, orthopedics, neurosurgery).

Treatments for Upper Crossed Syndrome and Costochondritis

▶ Pectoralis Major Stretch

- With the patient supine and the hands positioned under the head, gently stretch the elbows posteriorly to end point.

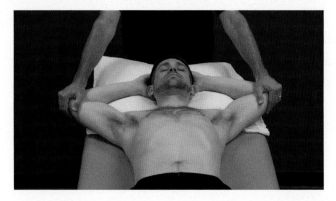

- Ask the patient to resist this stretch, using 10% effort, while taking three belly breaths. Then have the patient relax.
- Move the elbows further down to a new end point.
- Repeat these steps for a total of three stretch-relax cycles.

▶ Pectoralis Minor Stretch

- With the patient supine and the arms at the sides, place the heels of the clinician's hands between the distal clavicle and coracoid process.
- Stretch the coracoids down toward the table to the end point.
- Ask the patient to roll the shoulders forward, using 10% effort against resistance.

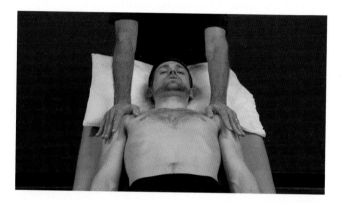

- Have the patient take belly breathes, then relax.
- Move the coracoids further down.
- Repeat these steps for a total of three stretch-relax cycles.

▶ Lateral Neck and Trapezius

- Have the patient side bend the neck away from the involved side and move the involved shoulder inferiorly.
- With one hand, hold the head in place. With your other hand, hold the shoulder down.

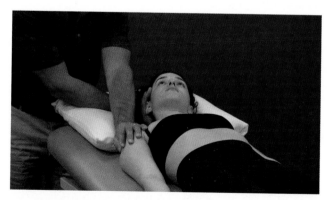

- Ask the patient to move the ear toward the shoulder with 10% effort against resistance while taking three belly breaths, then relax.
- Move the head and shoulder further apart. Repeat for total of three cycles.

⊙ Levator Scapulae

- With the patient standing, move the involved arm posteriorly and medially.
- Ask the patient to side flex the neck away from the involved side, rotate away from the affected side, and forward flex the neck to the end point (like trying to look at their hip).
- Ask the patient to hold their head in place with the uninvolved hand.
- Place your hand on the involved shoulder to stabilize.

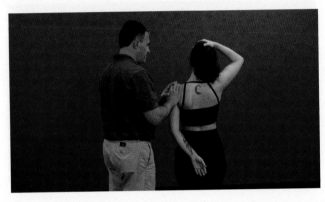

- Have the patient try to bring the ear toward the involved shoulder with 10% effort while taking three belly breaths. Then relax.
- Take up the slack in the neck and repeat these steps for a total of three cycles.

⊙ Kinesiology Taping for Upper Crossed Syndrome and Costochondritis

- Measure two strips of tape from the mid-trapezius region to below the opposite scapula.
- Apply the first 2 inches without tension over the mid-trapezius, diagonally across the back.
- Stretch the middle of the tape 25% to 50%, and apply it across the spine, ending just below the medial aspect of scapula.
- Apply the last 2 inches without any tension.
- Repeat these steps on the opposite side with the second piece of tape.
- Rub the tape to activate it.

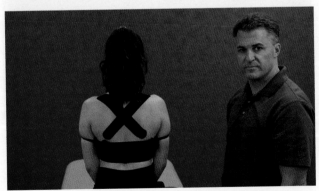

▶ Treatment for First Rib Syndrome

- With the patient supine and the head supported, rotate and side bend their head away from the involved side.
- Place your hand over the trapezius, with your thumb or a tennis or lacrosse-sized ball resting on the first rib.

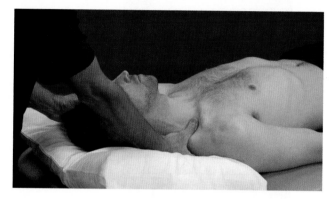

- While applying pressure inferiorly and medially to the first rib, ask the patient to take 10 belly breaths.
- Rotate and side bend the head toward the involved side, and repeat.

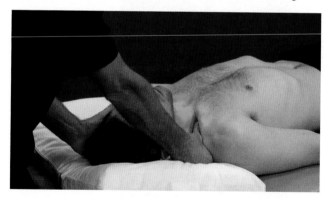

- Place the patient's opposite hand on the involved shoulder.
- Grasp the elbow and gently pull caudally.
- Gently press the first rib inferiorly and medially while the patient takes three belly breaths.

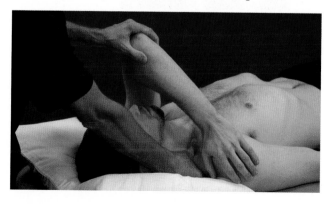

Treatment Summary

Upper Crossed Syndrome and Costochondritis

Pectoralis Major Stretch

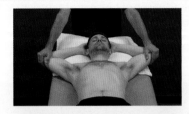

Pectoralis Minor Stretch

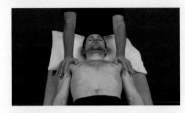

Lateral Neck and Trapezius Stretch

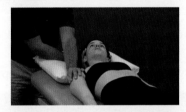

Levator Scapulae

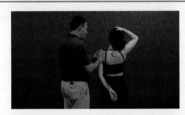

Kinesiology Taping for Upper Crossed Syndrome and Costochondritis

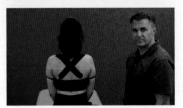

First Rib Syndrome

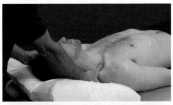
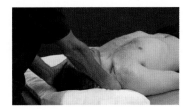
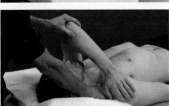

Sample Procedure Notes and Coding

Procedure	**E/M:** 99213 or 99214 **ICD 10:** Chest Pain: R07.9 Upper Crossed (Abnormal Posture): R29.3 First Rib Syndrome: Q76.5 **CPT:** 97140 – Manual therapy techniques one or more regions	
	Minutes	Units Reported
	8-22	1
	23-37	2
	38-52	3
	53-67	4
	--99070 – Supplies and Materials: applied by health care professional (list supplies/materials used)	
Informed Consent	After explaining the risks, benefits, and alternatives for the treatment, the patient gave verbal consent for the procedure	
Description of Procedure		
Outcomes/ Complications	The patient's symptoms reduced by ____% and there were no complications	
Instructions to Patient		
Time	Total time spent in **constant attendance** with the patient performing manual therapies: ____ minutes	

Note: If any of these exercises causes numbness or tingling, stop performing them and notify your clinician.

Shoulder Range of Motion

- Stand up straight, keep your head still, and squeeze your shoulder blades together.
- Hold this position for 5 seconds.
- Repeat these steps 10 times.

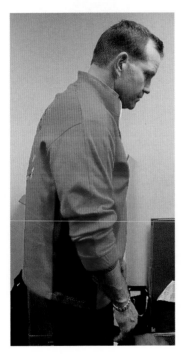 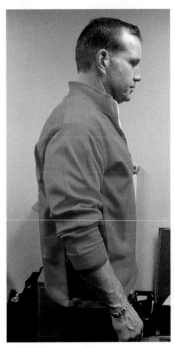

Rows (Isometric Scapular Engagement)

- Stand up straight and keep your head centered over your shoulders.
- Bend your elbows forward.
- Pull your elbows back and squeeze your shoulder blades together.
- Hold this position for 5 seconds.
- Repeat these steps 10 times.

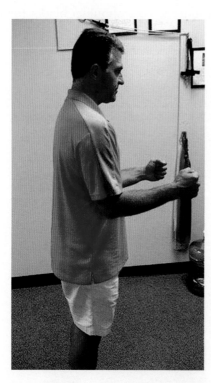 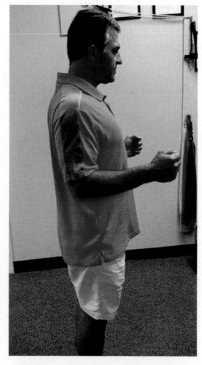

Wall and Neck Stretch

- Place your palm on the wall behind you with your elbow straight.
- Move your body toward the wall, feeling a stretch in your shoulder and chest.

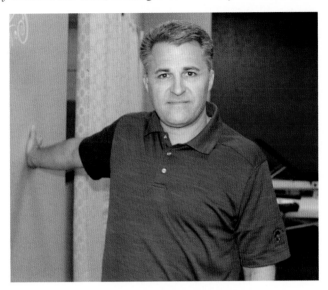

- Lean your head away from the wall and grasp the top of your head with your other hand.
- Gently pull your head away from the wall, increasing stretch in your neck.

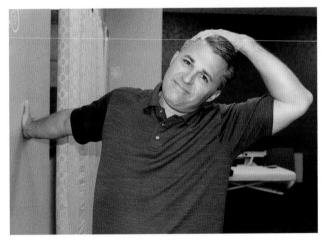

- Repeat the above-mentioned steps on the other side.

Bilateral Doorway (Pectoralis/Anterior Capsule) Stretch

- Stand in an open doorway, placing your hands on either side of the door jam.
- Place the leg of the affected side forward through the door.
- While keeping the spine straight, lean into doorway.
- Take three belly breaths, relax, and repeat 10 times.

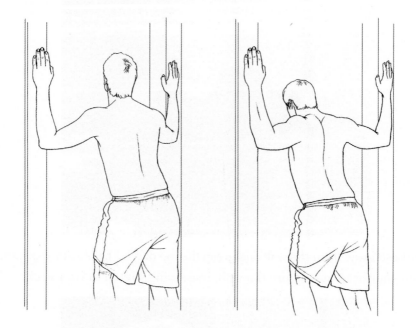

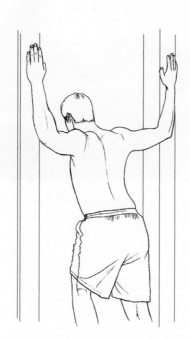

Stretch With Dowel

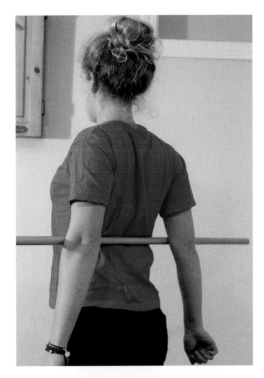

- While standing, hold a dowel behind your back with your elbows.
- Slowly turn your upper body to each side while keeping your hips facing forward.
- Take three belly breathes, then relax and turn to the opposite side.
- Repeat these steps 10 times in each direction.

Stretching Strap

- Position the strap behind you, grasping it in each hand with your palms facing forward.
- Pull your hands away from the lower back, taking three to five deep belly breaths.
- Relax and repeat for three cycles.

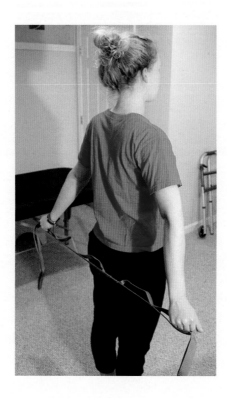

Subscapularis Stretching Strap

- Hold the strap in front of you with the pain-free hand and place the strap over the pain-free shoulder, letting the strap hang behind your back.
- Place your sore arm behind your back and grasp the strap.

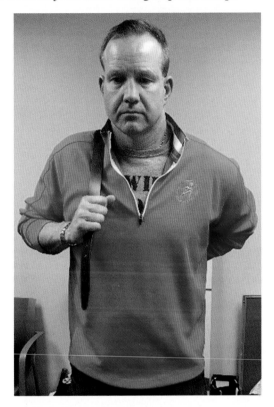

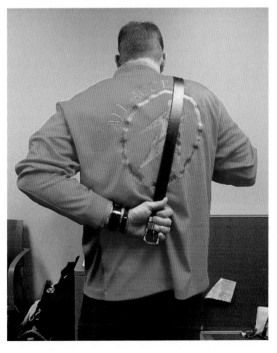

- Stand up straight; with your good arm, pull the strap down in front, which will pull the sore arm toward the middle and your hand up, stretching your shoulder.

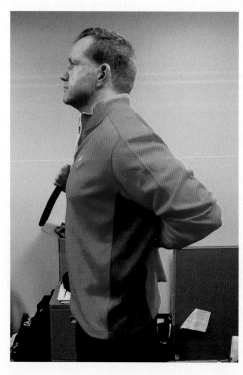

Levator Scapulae Self-Stretch

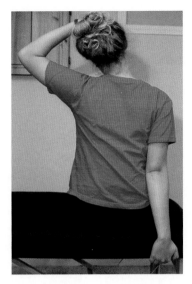

- Sit on a table or chair that allows you to grab behind you with the involved arm (as shown).
- Using the other arm, reach over and grab the side of your head and gently pull your ear toward your shoulder until you feel a gentle stretch.
- Hold this position and take three deep breaths, then relax and repeat three times.

Ball Stretch

- Place a tennis ball on a tender just to the side of your spine.
- Extend you arm.
- While pressing your back into the ball, move your extended arm up slowly over your head and back to your side 10 times.

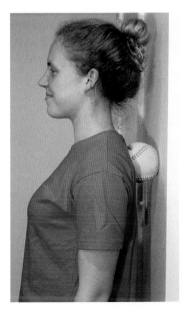

Stretching Strap Exercises

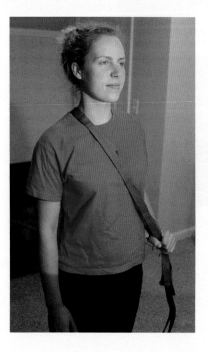 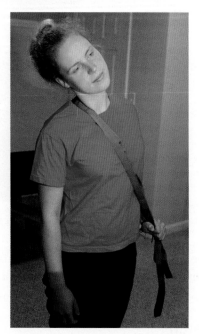

- Place the stretching strap at the bottom of your neck and over the first rib.
- Hold both ends tightly in the opposite hand.
- Lean your head toward the side that hurts and pull the straps down and away from the painful side while taking 10 belly breaths. Then relax.
- Reapply the strap, turning your head toward the side that hurts and this time moving your arm straight up in front of you with your palm facing sideways to over your head 10 times.
- When you are able to do these stretches without pain, remove the strap and place a tennis or lacrosse ball over the area of the first rib and again move your arm straight up in front of you with your palm facing sideways to over your head 10 times.

Patient Resource: Proper Positioning at Your Desk

- Ensure your desk, chair, and monitor are at eye level and that your mid-back is supported.
- Your elbows, hips, and knees should be positioned at 90 degrees, with the knees positioned slightly lower than the hips.
- If necessary, use a footstool.

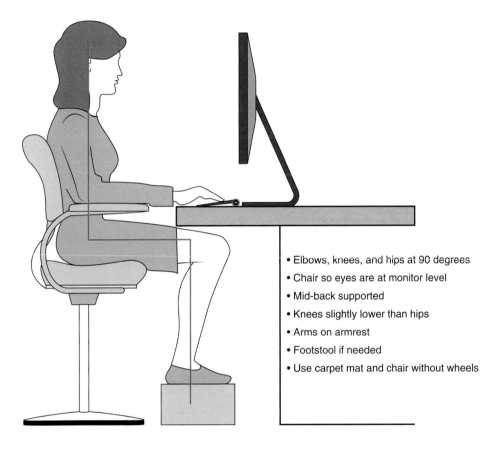

- Elbows, knees, and hips at 90 degrees
- Chair so eyes are at monitor level
- Mid-back supported
- Knees slightly lower than hips
- Arms on armrest
- Footstool if needed
- Use carpet mat and chair without wheels

Selected References

Foley CM, Sugimoto D, Mooney, D, Meehan, WP 3rd, Stracciolini A. Diagnosis and treatment of slipping rib syndrome. *Clin J Sport Med*. 2019;29(1):18-23.

Germanovich A, Ferrante, FM. Multi-modal treatment approach to painful rib syndrome: Case series and review of the literature. *Pain Physician*. 2016;19(3):E465-E4671.

CHAPTER | 9

ARM, ELBOW, AND WRIST PAIN

Falls and overuse plague the lower arms. Although mindfulness and attention are needed to lower the risk of falls, proper posture and form can help prevent and, when inflamed, treat the symptoms related to overuse. The financial and personal costs of treating carpal tunnel syndrome alone makes successful care of the lower arm, including the elbow and wrist, a critical component of clinical practice. Simple interventions can improve outcomes by simply applied nonsurgical treatment.

ELBOW PAIN

Differential Diagnosis

- Lateral or medial epicondylitis
- Pronator teres syndrome (tenderness or decreased ability to supinate, with referred symptoms of median nerve compression)
- Cubital tunnel syndrome (ulnar nerve impingement)
- Shoulder impingement
- Angina (left-sided)
- Cervical radiculopathy

Physical Examination

- Palpate and percuss to identify areas of discomfort (lateral epicondyle, medial epicondyle, pronator teres). (Figure 9-1) If you cannot palpate the area of discomfort, consider the etiology referred pain.

🛑 **ALERT:** Referred pain can be due to angina (left arm), cervical radiculopathy, shoulder impingement syndrome, and cubital tunnel syndrome.

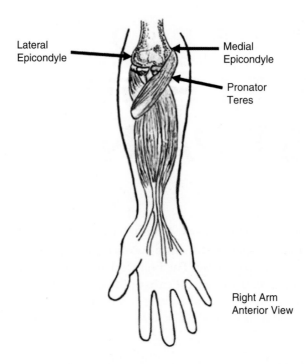

Lateral
Epicondyle

Medial
Epicondyle

Pronator
Teres

Right Arm
Anterior View

Figure 9-1 • Right arm, anterior view.

Diagnosis

- **Medial epicondylitis (Golfer's elbow):** Pain to palpation and percussion over medial epicondyle, made worse with extended elbow and resisted wrist flexion and/or pronation.
- **Lateral epicondylitis (Tennis elbow):** Pain to palpation and percussion over lateral epicondyle, made worse with extended elbow and resisted wrist extension and/or supination.
- **Pronator teres syndrome:** Tenderness over pronator teres muscle; compression at this site may cause pain or paresthesias radiating to the palm and/or digits within 30 seconds of compression; can mimic carpal tunnel syndrome; pain with supination and numbness over the anterior wrist and thenar eminence.

Physical Examination for Pronator Teres Syndrome

- The patient holds the elbow in 90 degrees of flexion and is asked to keep the elbow relaxed.
- The clinician holds the elbow to stabilize and grasps the patient's lower arm.
- The patient attempts to pronate their forearm as the clinician holds resistance (forcing the patient to contract pronator teres) and extends the elbow (Figure 9-2).
- If the patient's symptoms are reproduced, the median nerve is likely being compressed by the pronator teres.

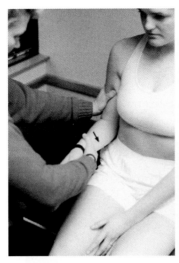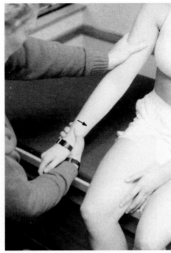

Figure 9-2 • Tests for pronator teres syndrome. (Reprinted from Palmer ML, Epler M. *Fundamentals of Musculoskeletal Assessment Techniques*. 2nd ed. Philadelphia: Wolters Kluwer; 1998 with permission.)

- **Cubital tunnel syndrome:** Impingement of the ulnar nerve as it traverses the medial elbow; often due to sleeping with elbow bent, leaning forward on elbows, cell phone use (called "cell phone elbow"), or trauma; symptoms include waking from sleeping with numbness and tingling over fourth and fifth digits with decreased grip strength

---

Remember the Rules
1. Move to a position of less pain and apply trigger point care
2. Stretch the SHORTENED muscle
3. Treat the region (above and below the pain)
4. Tape to support neutral position
5. Support definitive treatment (physical therapy, orthopedics, neurosurgery)

Treatment
⏵ Forearm Mobilization (for all forearm symptoms)

- With the patient's wrist in neutral (not flexed) and their arm supported by your thigh, place pressure downward and gently rock to the patient's tolerance on the patient's flexor tendons in the forearm to loosen adhesions of the tendon along the tendon sheath, from distal to proximal.

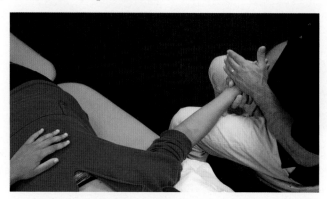

- Repeat 10 times and assess for patient response.

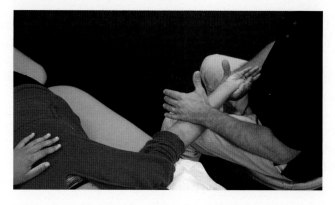

▶ Treatment for Lateral Epicondylitis and Pronator Teres Syndrome

This treatment is as effective as corticosteroid injection for lateral epicondylitis.
- Use your hand to stabilize the patient's elbow.

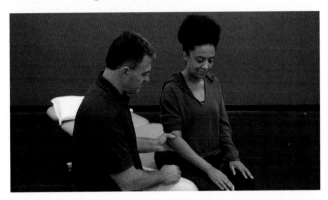

- Supinate the patient's hand with your other hand until the endpoint is reached.

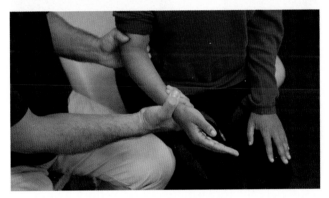

- Ask the patient to pronate the forearm against your resistance, using 10% effort.
- Have the patient take three belly breaths, then relax.
- As the patient relaxes, supinate to a new endpoint.

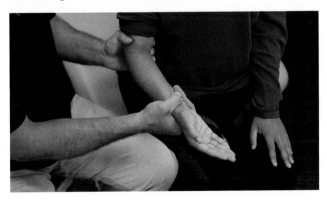

- Repeat these steps for a total of three cycles.

▶ Treatment for Medial Epicondylitis

- Stabilize the patient's elbow with your hand.

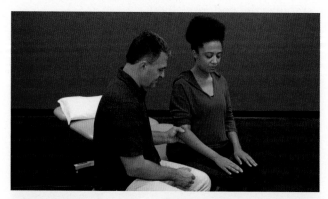

- Pronate the patient's hand with your other hand until the endpoint is reached.

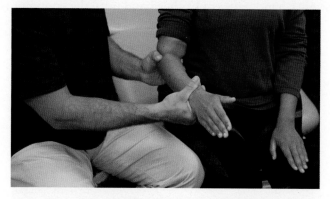

- Ask the patient to supinate the forearm, using 10% effort, against your resistance for three belly breaths, then relax.
- Pronate to new endpoint.

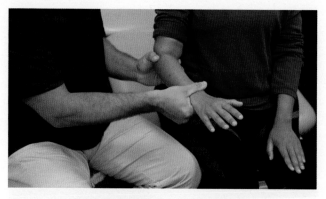

- Repeat these steps for a total of three cycles.

Cubital Tunnel Syndrome

- Massage the medial aspect of proximal forearm to relax muscles. Do not massage over the cubital tunnel or nerve.
- With their elbow wrist and fingers extended and their palm pointing away ("stop" gesture), ask the patient to gently flex and extend their wrist 10 times; if no symptoms, have them make a fist and repeat.

Treatment

- Have the patient keep the elbow straight and extend their wrist and fingers.

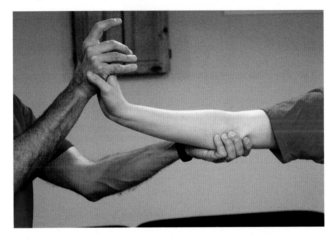

- With one hand supporting their and the other on the fingers, and forearm, hold resistance while asking the patient to flex their wrist, using 10% effort and take three belly breaths, then relax.
- As the patient relaxes, move the wrist into further extension.
- Repeat for three stretch-relax cycles.

WRIST PAIN

Differential Diagnosis

- Carpal tunnel syndrome
- Wrist sprain
- Bone dislocation
- Osteoarthritis

History and Diagnosis

- **Carpal tunnel syndrome:** Waking with numbness over median nerve distribution (Figure 9-3) in hand/wrist (anterior thumb, index, middle, and fourth fingers, in contrast to cubital tunnel syndrome, which causes numbness over fingers 4 and 5), thenar wasting, and weakened grip strength

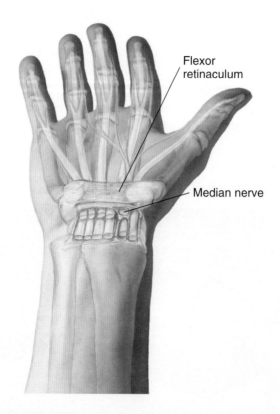

Flexor
retinaculum

Median nerve

Figure 9-3 • Anatomy of the wrist. (Reprinted from Clay JH, Allen L, Pounds DM. *Clay & Pounds' Basic Clinical Massage Therapy*. 3rd ed. Baltimore: Wolters Kluwer; 2015, with permission.)

Treatment
▶ Wrist Mobilization

• Place your thumbs over the midline of the wrist.

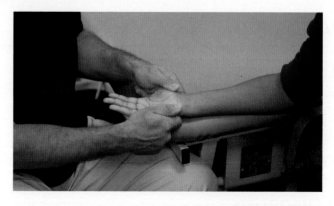

- Extend the wrist and massage the flexor retinaculum.
- Extend the wrist and massage the palmar aponeurosis.

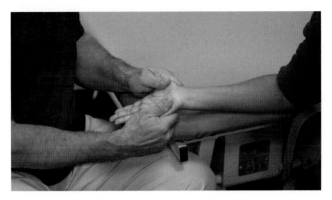

▶ Wrist Traction with Mobilization into Flexion or Extension

- Hold the patient's wrist at the distal aspect of the ulna and radius with one hand.
- Hold the patient's hand with your other hand.

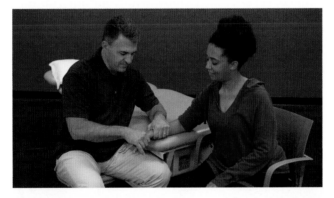

- Gently apply traction force.

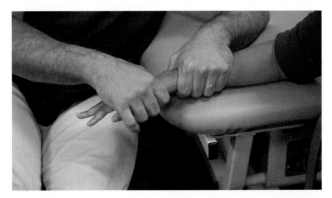

- While maintaining the traction force, gently move the patient's hand into flexion and extension for 10 repetitions.

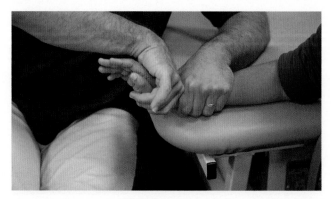

- The movement should be pain-free, with the goal of increasing the pain-free range of motion.

▶ Flossing for Carpal Tunnel Syndrome

- With the patient supine, support their elbow with your anterior thigh.

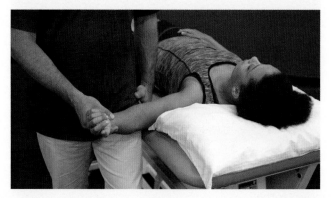

- Have the patient flex the elbow and flex the wrist while side-bending the head away from the involved side.
- *Passively* extend the elbow and then move the wrist into extension.

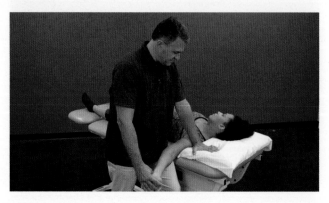

- Have the patient take three belly breaths, relax, and move the elbow and wrist back into flexion.
- Repeat these steps for a total of three cycles.
- This treatment may be as effective as surgery for women.
- If the patient does not improve, consider using the anterior neck stretch (see Chapter 6).

⊙ Kinesiology Taping for Lateral Epicondylitis

- Flex the patient's wrist and extend the elbow, with the fingers down.

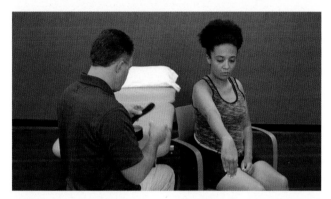

- Measure and cut two strips: one measured from above the epicondyle, over the epicondyle, and down to just proximal to the wrist, and the second about 5 inches long.
- Round all corners of the tape.
- Tear a 2-inch end of tape and apply it about 2" above epicondyle without tension.
- Apply a 50% stretch to the middle portion of the tape; then apply it over the involved epicondyle and down the length of the involved forearm.
- Apply the last 2 inches of tape without tension.

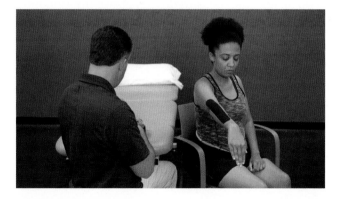

- Rub the tape to activate it.
- With the patient maintaining this position, apply the second piece of tape, with 50% tension, perpendicular to the involved epicondyle, applying the last 2 inches of each end without tension.

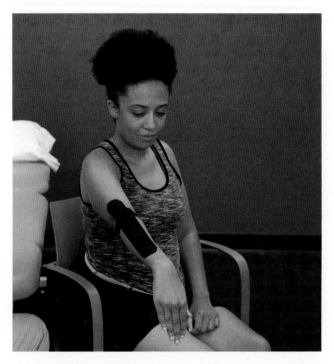

⊙ Kinesiology Taping for Medial Epicondylitis

- Flex the patient's wrist and extend the elbow, with the fingers up.
- Measure and cut two strips: one measured from above the epicondyle, over the epicondyle, and down to just proximal to the wrist, and the second about 5 inches long.
- Round all corners of the tape.
- Tear a 2-inch end of tape and apply it about 2" above epicondyle without tension.
- Apply a 50% stretch to the middle portion of the tape; then apply it over the involved epicondyle and down the length of the involved forearm.
- Apply the last 2 inches of tape without tension.

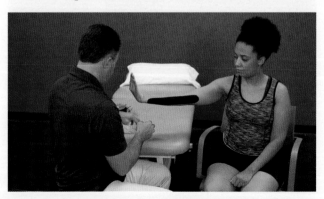

- With the patient maintaining this position, apply the second piece of tape, with 50% tension, perpendicular to the involved epicondyle, applying the last 2 inches on both ends without tension.

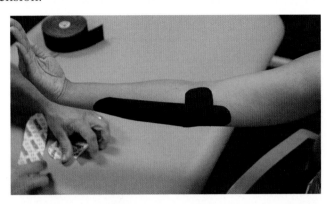

⏵ Kinesiology Taping for Pronator Teres Syndrome

- Start with the patient's elbow straight, the wrist extended, and fingers down.

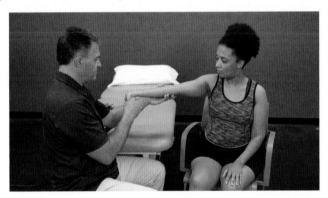

- Measure the tape from just proximal to the anterior wrist to up the arm and over the medial epicondyle to behind the elbow.

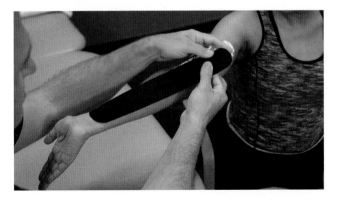

- Place 2" of tape just proximal to the wrist crease.
- Apply 50% stretch and move up the anterior forearm until 2" from antecubital fossa, then move the tape around the medial epicondyle, and flex the elbow to 90 degrees with the tape still under tension.
- Attach the tape under tension to just proximal to elbow posteriorly.
- Apply the last 2 inches without tension.

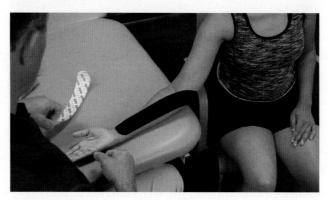

- Rub the tape to activate it.

Treatment Summary

Forearm Mobilization

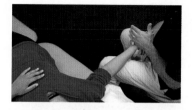 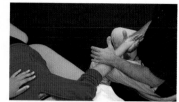

Treatment for Lateral Epicondylitis

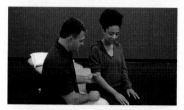 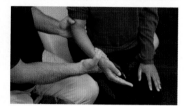

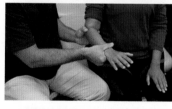

Treatment for Medial Epicondylitis

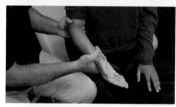 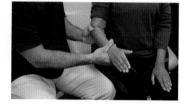

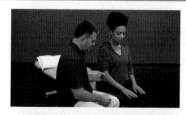

Cubital Tunnel Syndrome

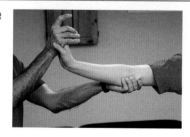

Wrist Mobilzation for Carpal Tunnel Syndrome

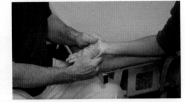 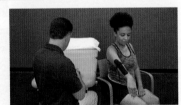

Wrist Traction with Mobilization into Flexion or Extension

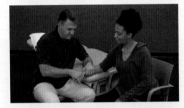 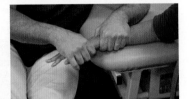

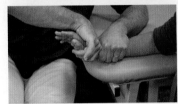

Flossing for Carpal Tunnel Syndrome

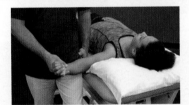 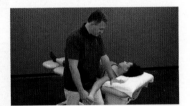

Kinesiology Taping for Lateral Epicondylitis

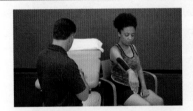 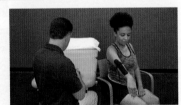

Kinesiology Taping for Medial Epicondylitis

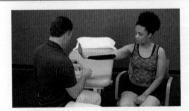 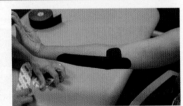

Kinesiology Taping for Pronator Teres Syndrome

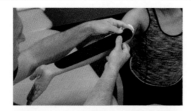
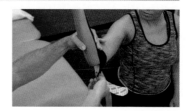
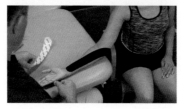

Sample Procedure Notes and Coding

Procedure	**ICD-10-CM Diagnosis Codes:**	
	Carpal Tunnel: G56.01 Medial Epicondylitis: M77.00 Lateral Epicondylitis: M77.10 Cubital Tunnel: G56.20 Elbow Pain: M25.52 **CPT:** 97140—Manual therapy techniques one or more regions	
	Minutes	Units Reported
	8-22	1
	23-37	2
	38-52	3
	53-67	4
	99070—Supplies and Materials: provided by the qualified health care professional over and above those usually included with the office visit (list supplies/materials used)	
Informed consent	After explaining the risks, benefits, and alternatives for the treatment, the patient gave verbal consent for the procedure.	
Description of Procedure		
Outcomes/ Complications	The patient's symptoms reduced by ___% and there were no complications.	
Instructions to Patient		
Time	Total time spent in **constant attendance** with the patient performing manual therapies: XX minutes	

Wrist Range of Motion

- Keeping your arm next to your body and your elbow bent, move your hand so your thumb is pointing forward

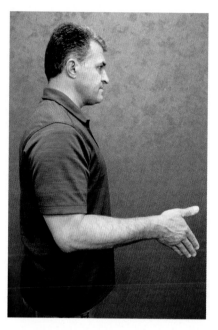

- Move your painful wrist so that your thumb points toward your head and then move it away. Do this movement for a total of 10 times

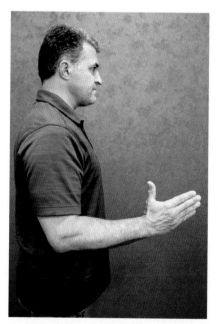

- If there is no pain with range of motion, hold a can of vegetables in your hand and GENTLY repeat the steps mentioned above.

Traction

- Bring your arm in front of you, palm toward the floor.
- Grab your wrist with your other hand and pull toward the opposite side.
- While pulling, move your painful wrist down (fingers pointing toward floor) and then up. Repeat 10 times.

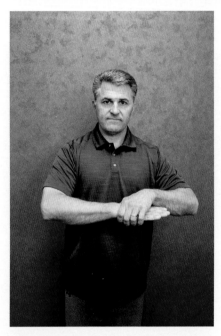

- Turn your arm so your palm faces your stomach, and while pulling, move your fingers toward your stomach, then opposite. Repeat 10 times.

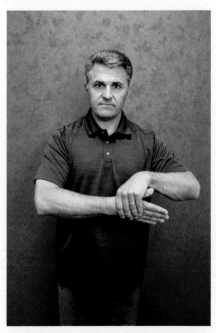

Resisted Flexion and Extension

- With your arm straight out, bend your wrist so your fingers point toward the floor.

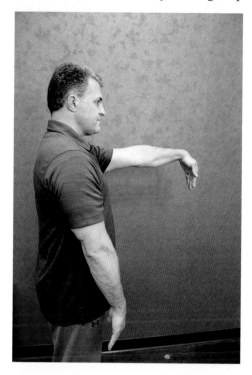

- Then, bend your wrist so your fingers point to the ceiling.

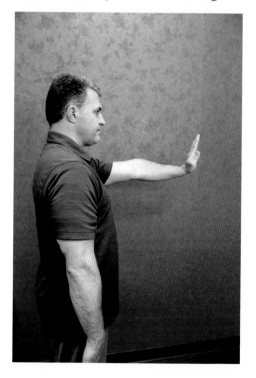

- Using your other hand, gently push your hand into further bending to gently stretch the muscles in your wrist and arm.

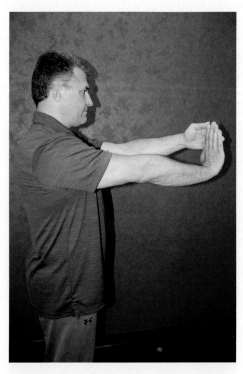

- Sleep with a wrist splint that prevents wrist flexion every night.

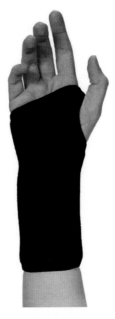

- Raise the computer screen at work so your head and shoulders are back and your elbows lay on the arm rests. Make sure your keyboard has a wrist support.

Patient Resource: Proper Positioning at Your Desk

- Ensure your desk, chair, and monitor are at eye level and that your mid-back is supported.
- Your elbows, hips, and knees should be positioned at 90 degrees, with the knees positioned slightly lower than the hips.
- If necessary, use a footstool.

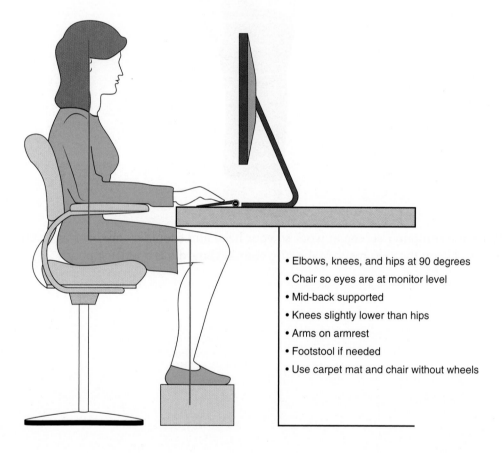

- Elbows, knees, and hips at 90 degrees
- Chair so eyes are at monitor level
- Mid-back supported
- Knees slightly lower than hips
- Arms on armrest
- Footstool if needed
- Use carpet mat and chair without wheels

- Apply a compression brace every morning before activities and take it off at the end of the day.
- For the strap to be effective, it must be put on properly. You may need two people at first to get the proper compression.

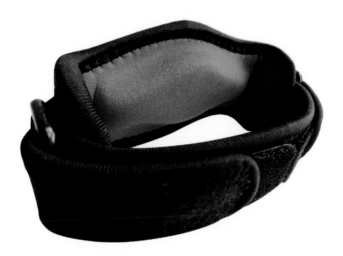

Applying an Epicondylitis Strap

- Move your arm out in front of you with the elbow straight.
- For lateral epicondylitis (outside elbow pain), point your palm toward the sky with your thumb pointing away from you.
- For medial epicondylitis (inside elbow pain), turn your arm so your thumb is pointing towards the sky.
- Position the strap BELOW the elbow (closer to the hand than the shoulder), with the pressure pad about 2" below the elbow joint.
- Tighten the strap so it is holding the area below the painful side, keeping muscles and tendons in place.

Selected References

Fernàndez-de-Las Peñas C, Ortega-Santiago R, de la Llave-Rincón AI, et al. Manual physical therapy versus surgery for carpal tunnel syndrome: a randomized parallel-group trial. *J Pain*. 2015;16(11):1087-1094.

Küçükşen S, Yilmaz H, Salli A, Uğurlu H. Muscle energy technique versus corticosteroid injection for management of chronic lateral epicondylitis: randomized controlled trial with 1-year follow-up. *Arch Phys Med Rehabil*. 2013;94:2068-2074.

CHAPTER | 1 0
ACUTE LOW BACK PAIN

Introduction

Acute low back pain treatment requires the practitioner to determine which motion or position decreases the patient's symptoms.

Lumbar radiculopathies are commonly due to nerve impingement by facet joint dysfunction, spasm of the piriformis muscle, and degenerative pathologies such as spinal stenosis. These symptoms often lessen when the patient is in a more flexed position, also called a *flexion bias*. When symptoms are due to lumbar disc dysfunction and protrusion, the patient's symptoms improve when they lean backward and extend the spine. This is called an *extension bias*.

The muscles involved in maintaining the lower back's stability include the psoas, quadratus lumborum, abdominal muscles, latissimus dorsi, paraspinal and oblique muscles (Figure 10-1). These muscles, often called "the core," contract to help stabilize the spine. When these muscles are appropriately engaged, they dissipate the stresses on the spine.

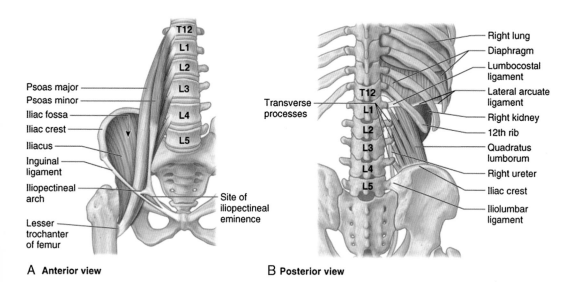

A **Anterior view**   B **Posterior view**

Figure 10-1 • Muscles involved in the lower back's stability. (Reprinted from Moore KL, Agur AM, Dalley F. *Essential Clinical Anatomy*. 5th ed. Baltimore: Wolters Kluwer; 2014 with permission.)

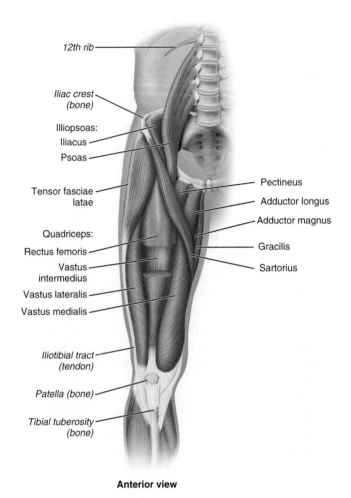

12th rib

Iliac crest (bone)

Illiopsoas:
Iliacus
Psoas

Tensor fasciae latae

Quadriceps:
Rectus femoris
Vastus intermedius
Vastus lateralis
Vastus medialis

Iliotibial tract (tendon)

Patella (bone)

Tibial tuberosity (bone)

Pectineus

Adductor longus

Adductor magnus

Gracilis

Sartorius

Anterior view

Figure 10-2 • Muscles of the hip that can contribute to back pain. (Reprinted from Archer PA, Nelson LA. *Applied Anatomy & Physiology for Manual Therapists*. Baltimore: Wolters Kluwer; 2012 with permission.)

Improving range of motion of these muscles and the joints they serve is referred to as *joint mobilization*. Providing manual techniques to joints with limited movement promotes joint mobilization, decreases pain, and improves range of motion.

Dysfunction of other muscle groups that contribute to supporting the back can also lead to back pain. Tightness of the muscles of the hip (iliacus, piriformis, rectus femoris) can cause back pain and sciatica (Figure 10-2). Weakness of the core muscles, such as the abdominal muscles and obliques, may cause instability around the spine and lead to pain symptoms.

The goal of treating acute low back pain is to move the patient to a posture that reduces their pain and helps regain conscious control of their core muscles.

Alert: In all patients with acute low back pain, please review and consider the Red Flags of acute low back pain for worrisome pathology (Box 10-1).

Box 10-1   Rule Out Red Flags

In patients who:
- are younger than 18 years or older than 50 years,
- with fever,
- weight loss,
- recent trauma,
- urinary incontinence,
- perineal anesthesia or
- history of cancer,

   consider a full evaluation to rule out conditions such as bone disease, tumor, and infection. This includes complete blood count with differential; a metabolic profile, alkaline phosphatase; erythrocyte sedimentation rate or C-reactive protein; plain films of the lumbosacral spine; or, if urinary or bowel incontinence is present, urgent neurosurgery referral.

Physical Examination

- Palpate bony structures for point tenderness, palpate muscles for spasm and trigger points, check patellar reflexes for symmetry, and have the patient plantar and dorsiflex the foot against resistance.
- Determine the position that **decreases** the patient's pain.
  - **Forward flexion bias:** Sitting and leaning forward reduces symptoms.
    - Common causes: piriformis spasm, degenerative disease such as spinal stenosis.
    - The lumbar spine is often flattened to maintain posture and reduce pain (Figure 10-3A).
    - Goal of treatment: Increase the patient's ability to flex forward by stretching the posterior muscle groups of the back and lengthening the hamstrings.
  - **Backward extension bias:** Standing and/or lying prone reduces symptoms.
    - Common causes: disc bulging or herniation.
    - The lumbar spine commonly has an exaggerated lordosis (concavity) (Figure 10-3B).
    - Goal of treatment: Increase the patient's ability to extend their back by lengthening their hip flexors.

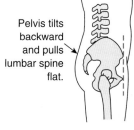
Pelvis tilts backward and pulls lumbar spine flat.

Normal

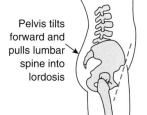
Pelvis tilts forward and pulls lumbar spine into lordosis

Extension Bias

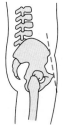
Flexion Bias

Figure 10-3 • Flexion and extension bias versus neutral back.

▶ Range-of-Motion Testing

- While standing, have patient put their hands on the anterior thighs for support and slowly forward flex. (If the patient cannot do this standing, have them sit.)

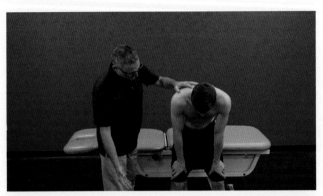

- Ask the patient how the pain changes from upright to forward flexed.

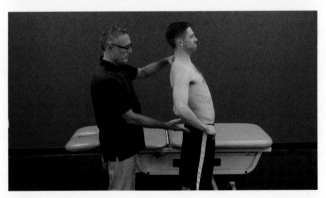

- Have the patient put the hands on the hips and extend the back, moving the back and shoulders posteriorly.
- Ask the patient how the pain changes from upright to extension.
- With the patient's hands relaxed at their sides, have the patient side bend to one side, then the other, asking how the pain changes based on each side.

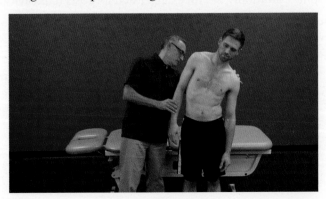

Treatment

- Treatment is based on bias.

> **Remember the Rules**
> **1.** Move to a position of less pain and apply trigger point care.
> **2.** Stretch the SHORTENED muscle.
> **3.** Treat the region (above and below pain).
> **4.** Tape to support neutral position.
> **5.** Support definitive treatment (physical therapy, orthopedics, neurosurgery).

Techniques for Flexion Bias (Forward Flexion Reduces Pain)

- These techniques are for when a patient prefers for their low back to be in a state of flexion.
- Patients with flexion bias may be more comfortable sitting than standing and tend to lean forward when they go to stand or walk.
- Goal of treatment is to increase joint and muscle range of motion in flexion; muscles to stretch include paraspinal muscles of the back and hamstrings.

▶ Cannonball

- Have the patient lie supine and pull the knee on the affected side up to chest as far as able and then place their foot under your arm.

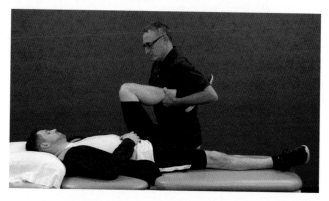

- The clinician grasps their mid-calf in one hand and around their knee with the other.
- Move the knee toward the axilla on the involved side to the limit.
- Have the patient attempt to extend the leg using 10% effort against resistance while taking three belly breaths and then relax.
- Move the patient's knee into greater hip flexion and repeat the above-mentioned steps for a total of three stretch-relax cycles.

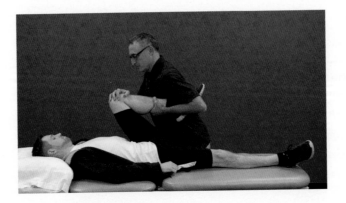

▶ Assisted Posterior Pelvic Tilt

- With the patient supine, flex the hip and knee, placing the knee over your shoulder.

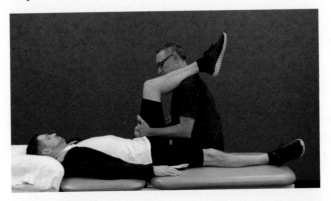

- Pull the patient's proximal thigh toward the clinician and ask the patient to try to bring the leg back to the table using 10% effort while taking three belly breaths.
- As the patient relaxes, move the hip into increased flexion.

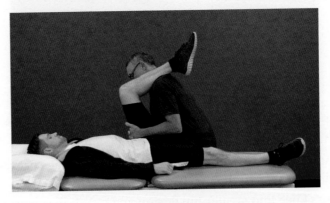

- Repeat these steps for a total of three stretch-relax cycles.

▶ Straight-Leg Raise With Traction

- Have the patient lie on a lowered table. Alternatively, the clinician stands on a step stool.
- Assist the patient to raise the straightened leg to 45 degrees.
- Grasp the ankle and provide a caudal traction (away from the hip) while the patient takes three belly breaths, then relaxes.

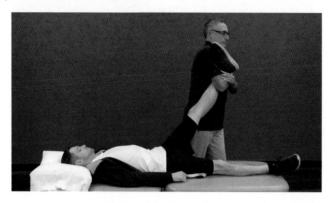

- Increase hip flexion and repeat these steps for a total of three stretch-relax cycles.

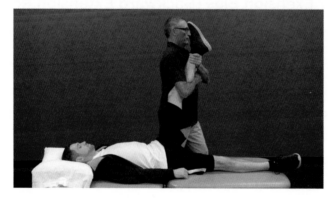

▶ Hamstring Stretch

- Have the patient flex the hip and knee to 90/90 position.

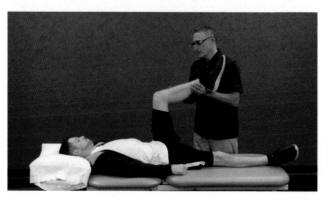

- Grasp the patient's thigh just proximal to the knee and at the ankle.

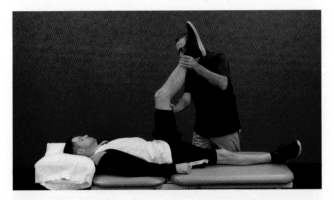

- Assist the patient in extending the knee until it is maximally stretched.
- Ask the patient to use 10% effort to push the heel down into your shoulder or hand while taking three belly breaths.
- Have the patient relax while you move the knee into further extension.
- Repeat these steps for a total of three stretch-relax cycles.

Techniques for Exension Bias (Backward Extension Reduces Pain)

- These techniques are used when the patient's preferred position is with the spine straightened and an increased lordosis in the lower back.
- Patients tend to feel better standing than sitting.
- Symptoms are often correlated with herniated discs and/or tight hip flexors.
- Goal of treatment is to increase extension through joint mobilization and lengthening the hip flexors (quadriceps, psoas, and piriformis).

▶ Lumbar Glide

- Have the patient lie on their stomach. Palpate for a tender lumbar spinous process.

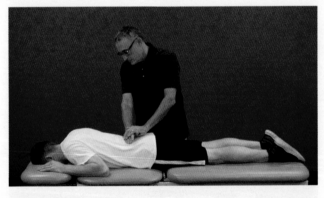

- Apply pressure downward (from posterior to anterior) to the lumbar spine while you direct the patient to move up onto their elbows. Hold for three belly breaths.

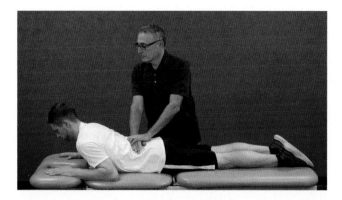

- Have the patient return to prone.
- Move your hands to the next tender spinous process area and repeat the process.

▶ Supine Psoas and Rectus Femoris Stretch

- Ask the patient to sit as close to the end of the table as possible.

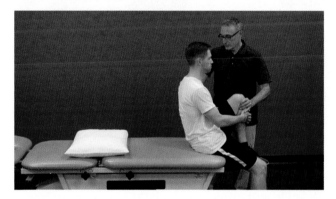

- Have the patient to flex the hip and knee on the uninvolved side and draw the knee toward the chest.
- With your assistance, have the patient lie supine on the table; this will leave the leg on the involved side hanging off the table.
- Stabilize the uninvolved knee with your chest and hold resistance against the involved knee toward the floor.

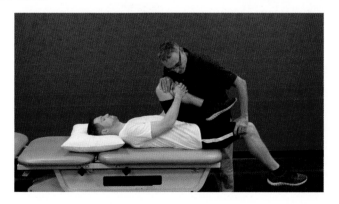

- Ask the patient to flex the involved hip, using 10% effort, and to take three belly breaths then relax.
- Move the involved hip into further extension.
- Repeat these steps for a total of three stretch-relax cycles.

▶ Prone Rectus Femoris and Psoas Stretch

- With the patient prone, flex the patient's knee while extending the hip to its limit.

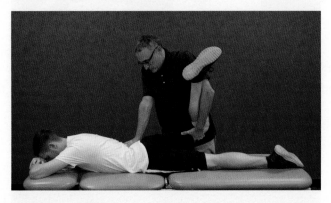

- Have the patient try, using 10% effort, to forward flex the hip against your resistance while taking three belly breaths.
- Have the patient relax while you move the leg into further extension.
- Follow these steps for a total of three stretch-relax cycles.

Leg Pull

- Have the patient perform a straight leg raise to 20 degrees.
- Grasp the patient's ankle and provide a caudal traction (away from the hip) while the patient takes three belly breaths, then relaxes.

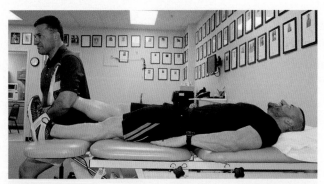

- If there is no discomfort with the leg pull, repeat these steps with gentle oscillations back and forth, while maintaining traction.

Hip Flexor Stretch

Supine

- With the patient supine, place the involved leg off the end of the table.
- Flex the patient's other hip and knee.
- Hold both knees stable and ask the patient to raise the involved knee against your resistance while taking three belly breathes, then relax; moving the involved leg further into extension.

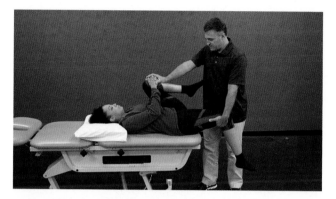

- Repeat these steps for three stretch-relax cycles.

Prone

- With the patient prone and involved knee flexed, lift the involved leg off the table to the end point.

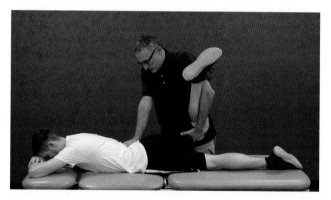

- Ask the patient to gently bring the knee down toward the table, using 10% effort, against resistance for three belly breaths.
- Have the patient relax and move the hip further into extension.
- Repeat these steps for total of three cycles.

Additional Syndromes and Treatment With Acute Low Back Pain

The quadratus lumborum is a deep muscle that can be the cause of acute low back pain or go into spasm to relieve the stress from other causes of back pain.

▶ Sitting Quadratus Lumborum Stretch: Reciprocal Inhibition Procedure

- Have the patient sit in an upright, relatively pain-free position and place the arm of the involved side on the side/top of their head.
- Ask the patient to side bend away from the pain to their limit.

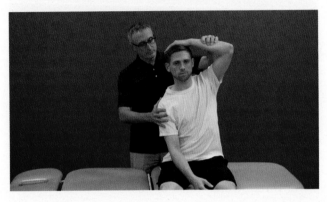

- Hold the patient's bent elbow or arm in one hand and their opposite shoulder in the other.
- Ask the patient to try and sit up straight with 10% effort, against your resistance.
- As the patient relaxes, further bend the patient away from the involved side.
- Repeat these steps for a total of three cycles.

▶ Side-lying Quadratus Lumborum Stretch

- Position the patient side-lying with the involved side up.
- Flex the uninvolved hip and knee forward, and move the involved leg posteriorly and off the side of table.
- Position the top arm above the patient's head.

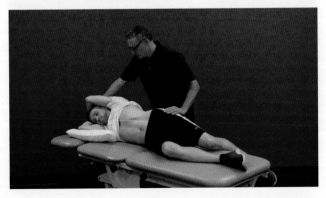

- Cross your hands, placing one on the anterior superior iliac spine and the other on the inferior aspects of the patient's ribs.

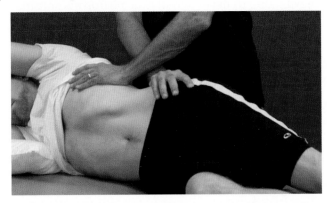

- Ask the patient to side bend, moving the hip up toward the ribs against your resistance, while taking three belly breaths.

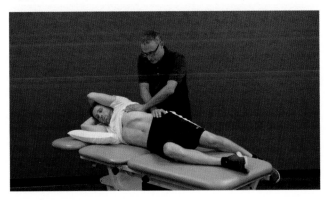

- As the patient relaxes, further stretch the side.
- Repeat the steps for a total of three stretch-relax cycles.

Treatments for Radiculopathy and Sciatica

- A radiculopathy may be due to herniated disc or piriformis spasm.
- Disc herniation-induced symptoms will often worsen when the torso is flexed and lessen when the back is extended.
- The piriformis may be the cause when the pain originates in the buttocks and then travels down the posterior thigh.
- In patients with radiculopathy and sciatica, attempt to treat piriformis syndrome.

⊙ Evaluating for Radiculopathies (Piriformis Syndrome)

- Have the patient lie down with the affected side up.
- Flex hip to 60 degrees.
- Place your upper hand on the hip and your lower hand on the knee.
- Holding the hip stable, push down on the knee, toward the floor.

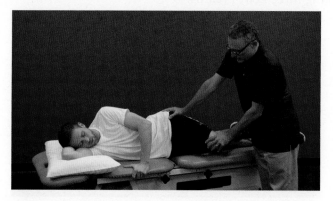

- If this action elicits pain, it is likely due to piriformis syndrome.
- Treatment can be best performed while in this position.

⊙ Side-lying Piriformis Stretch

- Have the patient side lie down with the affected side up.

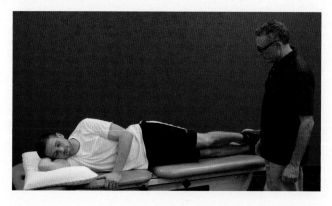

- Flex the involved hip to 60 degrees, letting the knee hang off the side of the table.
- Place your upper hand on the hip and your lower hand on the knee.

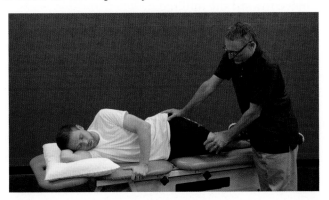

- Move the knee toward the floor to the limit.
- Hold resistance while the patient pushes the knee up against your hand, using 10% effort, taking three belly breaths and then relaxing.
- Move the knee further toward the floor (into further internal rotation).
- Repeat these steps for a total of three stretch-relax cycles.

Supine Piriformis Stretch

- With the patient supine, place a rolled towel in the patient's groin-hip flexor crease.

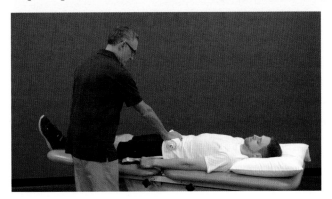

- Have the patient bring their flexed hip and knee across midline toward the opposite shoulder, keeping the involved posterior superior iliac spine on the table. Their involved foot will move toward the midline.

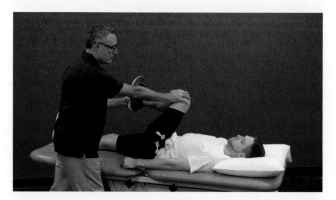

- At the patient's limit, hold resistance on the knee and ankle while the patient tries to move the knee laterally, using 10% effort and taking three belly breaths, then relaxing.

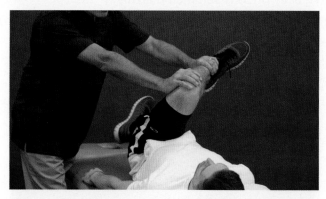

- As the patient relaxes, move the knee further toward the opposite axilla.
- Repeat these steps for a total of three stretch-relax cycles.

▶ Prone Piriformis Release

- With the patient prone, flex the involved knee to 90 degrees.

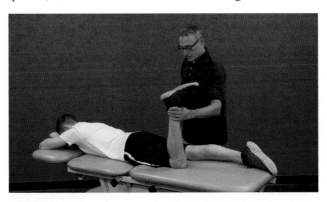

- Move the hip to external rotation (so the foot moves medially).
- Using a soft fist, apply pressure along the piriformis while moving the foot laterally to limit.

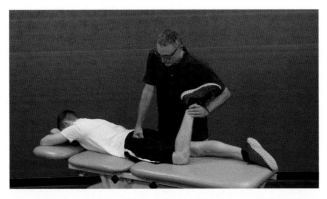

- Hold the ankle and ask the patient to move the foot medially, using 10% effort, against resistance while taking three belly breaths.
- As the patient relaxes, move the foot further laterally.

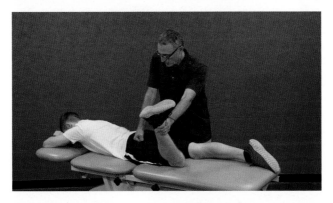

- Repeat these steps for a total of three stretch-relax cycles.

Kinesiology Taping

▶ **Kinesiology Taping for Back Pain**

- Have the patient bend slightly forward, resting their hands or elbows on a stable surface or the hands on the thighs to diminish the pain and the activation of spinal muscles.

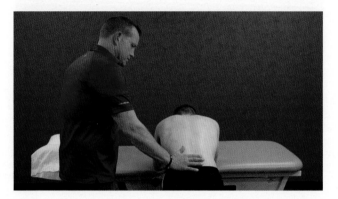

- Cut three pieces of tape approximately 12 to 14 inches in length.
- Trim off the corners of the ends of the tape to avoid edges getting caught on clothing.
- Tear the paper in the middle, and hold the ends with the backing still in place.
- Pull to 50% tension and apply horizontally in the region of pain; apply the ends of the tape with 0% tension.

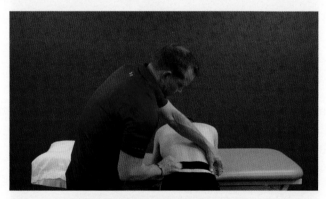

- Rub the tape vigorously to activate the tape's adhesive.

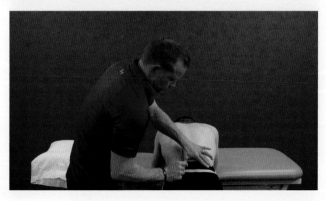

- Repeat the above-mentioned steps until you have taped into a star pattern over the area of maximal discomfort, as shown.

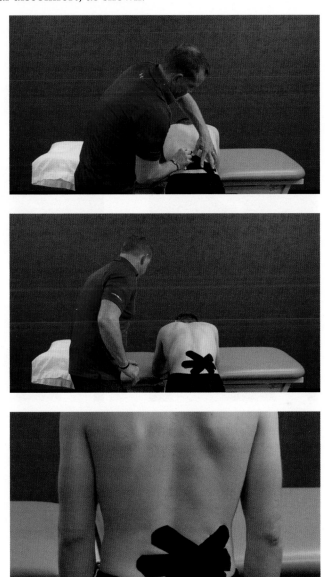

- Instruct the patient to leave the tape in place for 2 to 5 days or until the tape falls off.

Treatment Summary

Techniques for Flexion Bias: Forward Flexion Reduces Pain

Cannonball

Assisted Posterior Pelvic Tilt

Straight-Leg Raise with Traction

Hamstring Stretch

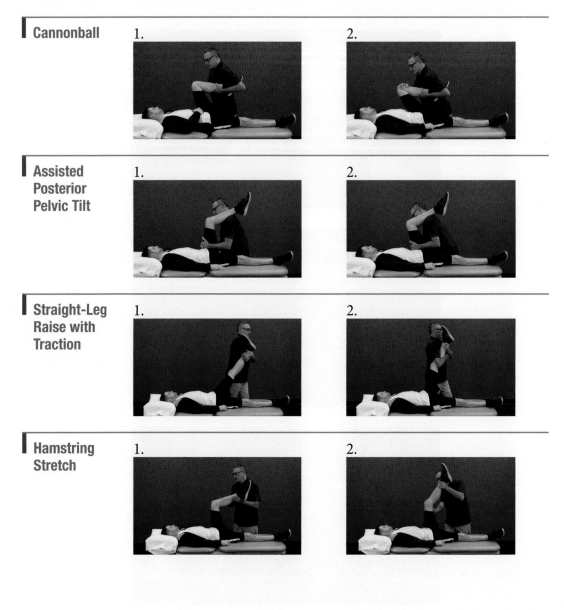

Techniques for Extension Bias: Backward Extension Reduces Pain

Lumbar Glide

1.
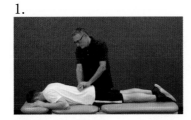

2.
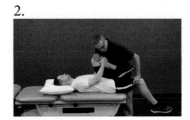

Supine Psoas and Rectus Femoris Stretch

1.
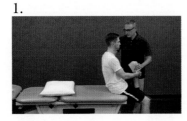

2.
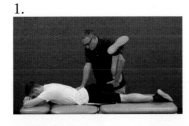

Prone Rectus Femoris and Psoas Stretch

1.
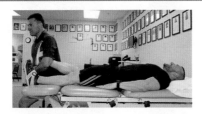

Leg Pull

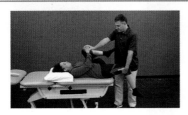

Hip Flexor Stretch

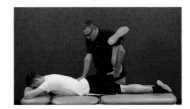

Additional Syndromes and Treatment Seen with Acute Low Back Pain

Sitting Quadratus Lumborum Stretch: Reciprocal Inhibition Procedure

1.
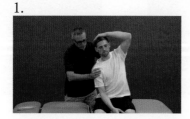

2.
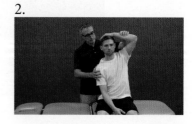

Side-Lying Quadratus Lumborum Stretch

1.
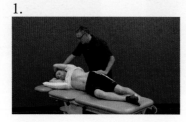

2.
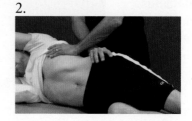

Treatments for Radiculopathy and Sciatica

Side-lying Piriformis Stretch

1.
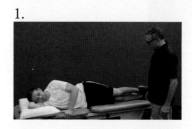

2.
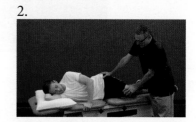

Supine Piriformis Stretch

1.
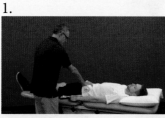

2.
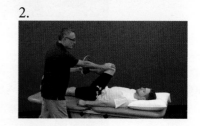

3.
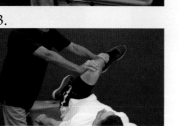

Prone Piriformis Release

1.
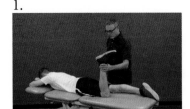

2.
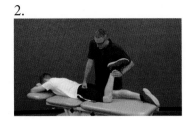

3.
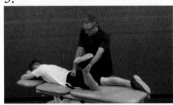

Kinesiology Taping

Kinesiology Taping for Back Pain

1.
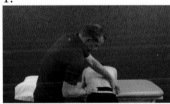

2.
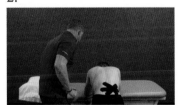

3.
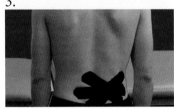

Sample Procedure Notes and Coding

Procedure:	CPT Codes 99140 x X units ICD-10-CM Diagnosis Code(s): **ICD-10-CM Diagnosis Codes:** 99213 or 99214 M54.5 Low Back Pain & Modifier 25 M54.16 Lumbar Radiculopathy **CPT:** 97140 – Manual therapy techniques one or more regions

Minutes	Units Reported
8-22	1
23-37	2
38-52	3
53-67	4

	99070 – Supplies and Materials: provided by the qualified health care professional over and above those usually included with the office visit (list supplies/materials used)
Informed Consent	After explaining the risks, benefits, and alternatives for the treatment, the patient gave verbal consent for the procedure
Description of Procedure	
Outcomes/Complications	__none; other:
Instructions to Patient	Reviewed and given Patient Education sheet for: __flexion bias __extension Bias __Piriformis Syndrome __Quadratus Lumborum __Refer to Physical Therapy
Time	Total time spent in **constant attendance** with the patient performing manual therapies: XX minutes

These exercises should be performed for a maximum of three times per day.

Stretching Strap or Dowel

Sitting

- Using a stretching strap or dowel, apply pressure at or above the area of pain.
- Pull the strap or dowel forward, and slowly forward bend while maintaining tension on the strap.
- Move the strap or dowel to get best pain-free forward flexion and repeat 10 times.

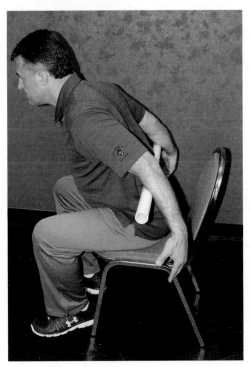

On Your Back

- Lie on your back with your head supported.
- Wrap the stretching strap under the arch of foot and, **using your hands**, pull your leg forward until you feel a pull behind your thigh.

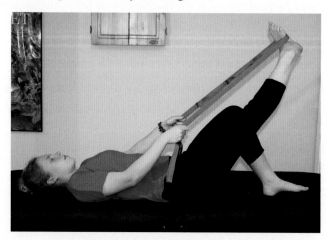

- Take three belly breaths, relax, and then try to move your leg further toward the ceiling

Hip Flexor and Hamstring Stretch

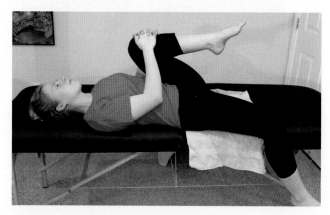

- Lie on bed and let affected leg hang off the side.
- Pull the unaffected leg toward the chest, pushing the small of your back into the bed.
- Hold this pose for 30 seconds.
- Repeat these steps three times.

Hook-Lying (90/90)/Isometric Posterior Pelvic Tilt

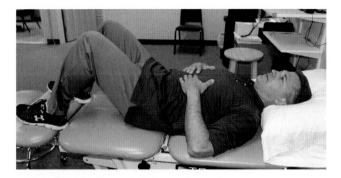

- Lie on your back and flex your knees and hips.
- Drive your heels down and squeeze, your buttocks and tighten your stomach (like you are about to get punched), using 10% effort, and hold for three belly breaths.
- Relax and repeat these steps 10 times.

Piriformis Stretch

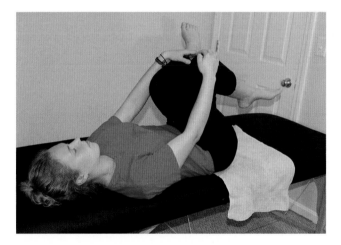

- Cross your knee on the painful side over the opposite thigh.
- Using your other leg or a stretching strap, pull the involved knee up toward your chest.
- Take three belly breaths and relax.
- Repeat these steps 5 to 10 times.

Basic Resting Stretch

- Rest with hips and knees flexed and perform belly breaths.

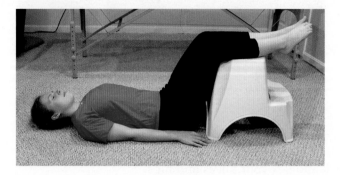

Repeat these exercises for a maximum of three times per day.

Stretching Strap or Dowel Stretch (Sitting)

- Place a stretching strap or dowel into your lower back/top of sacrum.
- Extend the back, then take three belly breaths.
- Repeat these steps 5 to 10 times.

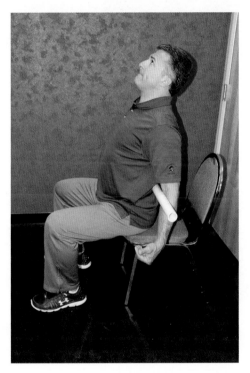

Gluteus Bridge

- Plant your feet on the floor with your knees bent.
- Raise your lower back off of the floor and hold for 3 to 5 seconds, then relax.
- Repeat these steps 5 to 10 times.

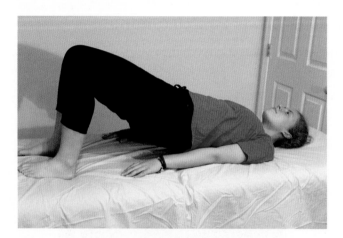

Stretching Strap on for Hip Flexors/Quadriceps

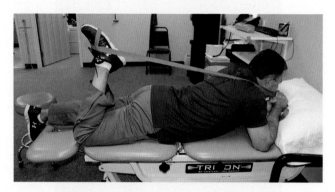

- Wrap the stretching strap around your ankle.
- Using stretching strap, pull your foot toward your head, keeping the hips stable.
- Using 10% effort, push your ankle into the strap and take three belly breaths.
- Relax while moving the foot closer to your head.
- Repeat these steps for a total of 5 to 10 stretch-relax cycles.

- If able, lie on your back in bed and place the stretching strap around your ankle.

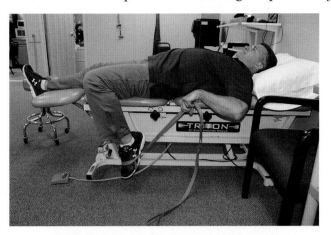

- Gently pull toward the head of the bed.
- Using 10% effort, push your foot into the strap and take three belly breaths, then relax, and pull your foot toward.
- Repeat these steps for a total of 5 to 10 stretch-relax cycles.

Positioning While Sleeping

- Sleep with pillows under your knees or lie on your stomach with a pillow under your chest.

- Sit with your legs apart.
- Place a pillow under your elbow on the affected side.

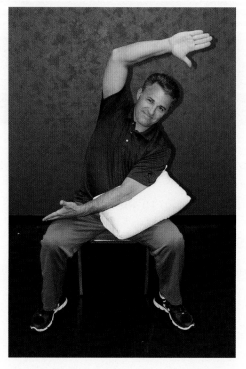

- Move the shoulder on the side that does not hurt down as far as possible and let your head lean toward the floor.
- Move the arm on the involved side up over your head and gently stretch.
- Take three belly breathes, then relax.
- Lean again away from the painful side, moving the top arm slowly up and over, reaching as far as possible, and take three belly breaths.
- To sit up, **push your elbow down on the pillow** to lift yourself up.

Selected References

Areeudomwong P, Wongrat W, Neammesri N, et al. A randomized controlled trial on the long-term effects of proprioceptive neuromuscular facilitation training, on pain-related outcomes and back muscle activity, in patients with chronic low back pain. *Musculoskeletal Care.* 2017;15(3):218-229.

Ay S, Konak HE, Evcik D, et al. The effectiveness of Kinesio Taping on pain and disability in cervical myofascial pain syndrome. *Rev Bras Reumatol Engl Ed.* 2017;57(2):93-99.

Day JM, Nitz AJ. The effect of muscle energy techniques on disability and pain scores in individuals with low back pain. *J Sport Rehabil.* 2012:194-198.

El-Abd AM, Ibrahim AR, El-Hafez HM. Efficacy of kinesio taping versus postural correction exercises on pain intensity and axioscapular muscles activation in mechanical neck dysfunction: a randomized blinded clinical trial. *J Sports Med Phys Fitness.* 2017;57(10):1311-1317.

Kelle B, Güzel R, Sakalli H. The effect of Kinesio taping application for acute non-specific low back pain: a randomized controlled clinical trial. *Clin Rehab.* 2015;30(10):997-1003.

KwwangYong Park MS, KyoChul S. The effects on the pain index and lumbar flexibility of obese patients with low back pain after PNF scapular and PNF pelvic patterns. *J Phys Ther Sci.* 2014;26(10):1571-1574.

Selkow NM, Grindstaff TL, Cross KM, et al. Short-term effect of muscle energy technique on pain in individuals with non-specific lumbopelvic pain: a pilot study. *J Man Manip Ther.* 2009;17(1):E14-E18.

Shih HS, Chen SS, Cheng SC, et al. Effects of Kinesio taping and exercise on forward head posture. *J Back Musculoskelet Rehabil.* 2017;30(4):725-733.

Tufo A, Desai GJ, Cox WJ. Psoas syndrome: a frequently missed diagnosis. *JAOA.* 2012;112(8):522-528.

Wilson E, Payton O, Donegan-Shoaf L, et al. Muscle energy technique in patients with acute low back pain: a pilot clinical trial. *J Orthop Sports Phys Ther.* 2003;33:502-512.

Ulger O, Demirel A, Oz M, et al. The effect of manual therapy and exercise in patients with chronic low back pain: double blind randomized controlled trial. *J Back Musculoskelet Rehabil.* 2017;30(6):1303-1309.

Figure Credit

Gluteus Bridge: Reprinted from Williams A. *Study Guide to Accompany Massage Mastery*: Theory and Technique. Baltimore: Wolters Kluwer; 2012 with permission.

CHAPTER | 11
UPPER LEG AND HIP

Introduction

Upper leg and hip pain may be due to referred pain from the lower back. Hip pain can also refer pain up to the lower back and down into the groin.

Differential Diagnosis

Differential diagnosis of muscular upper leg and hip pain includes:
- referred pain from the lower back,
- hip flexor dysfunction (psoas and iliacus [sometimes considered together as the iliopsoas] and rectus femorus),
- hip extensor dysfunction (hamstring/gluteals),
- adductor and abductor dysfunction,
- piriformis dysfunction
- disorders of the iliotibial (IT) band.
- Non-muscular causes include radiculopathies, SI dysfunction, bone disorders, and osteoarthritis, labral diseases of the hip (labral tears), bursitis, IT band dysfunction, and hernia (Figure 11-1).

Examination
Iliac Crest Height

- Assess the iliac crest height, comparing height from side to side.

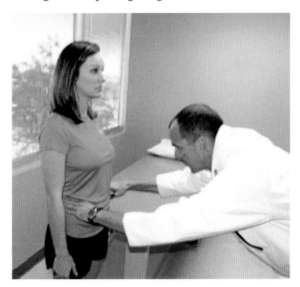

- If one sacroilial crest is higher on one side (and no scoliosis), perform a leg pull on that side.
  - Have the patient perform a straight leg raise to 20 degrees.
  - Grasp the patient's ankle and provide a caudal traction (away from the hip) while the patient takes three belly breaths, then relaxes.

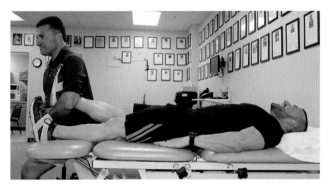

  - If there is no discomfort with the leg pull, repeat these steps with gentle oscillations back and forth, while maintaining traction.

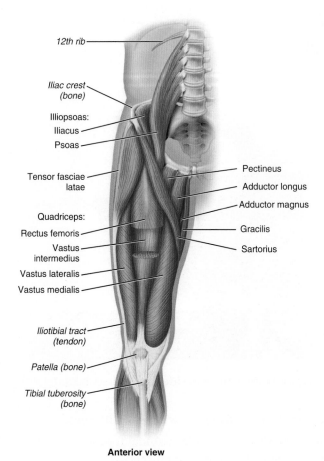

12th rib

Iliac crest (bone)

Illiopsoas:
Iliacus
Psoas

Tensor fasciae latae

Quadriceps:
Rectus femoris
Vastus intermedius
Vastus lateralis
Vastus medialis

Iliotibial tract (tendon)

Patella (bone)

Tibial tuberosity (bone)

Pectineus

Adductor longus

Adductor magnus

Gracilis

Sartorius

Anterior view

Figure 11-1 • Muscles of the hip complex. (Reprinted from Archer P, Nelson LA. *Applied Anatomy & Physiology for Manual Therapists*. Baltimore: Wolters Kluwer; 2012, with permission.)

▶ FABER (Flexion ABduction External Rotation) or Patrick Testing

- Tests the IT band, internal rotators, and hip flexors.
- Decreased range of motion or pain in the groin may imply a hip pathology (labral tear, osteoarthritis, adductor weakness/iliopsoas dysfunction, IT band, bursitis, hip flexors)
- If ROM induces symptoms, palpate painful region to locate etiology:
  - Anterior: hip flexors
  - Posterior: hip extenders (hamstrings, piriformis, gluteals)
  - Medial: adductors
  - Lateral: IT band or trochanteric bursitis
- If you cannot palpate the pain, consider hip joint derangement (osteoarthritis, labral dysfunction)

Performing the Test

- With the patient supine, the involved leg is placed with the hip flexed and abducted, and the lateral malleolus is moved to rest on the contralateral thigh just superior to the knee.

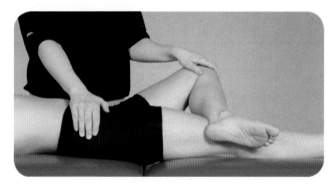

- While stabilizing the opposite pelvis at the anterior superior iliac spine (ASIS), a force is applied toward the table to the involved knee to further the hip's external rotation and abduction.
- If this induces pain, think hip joint disease (osteoarthritis, labral tear), iliopsoas spasm, or sacroiliac joint dysfunction.

- If this maneuver does NOT induce pain, move the leg into internal rotation, with the involved knee pointing toward the opposite shoulder, and apply pressure.

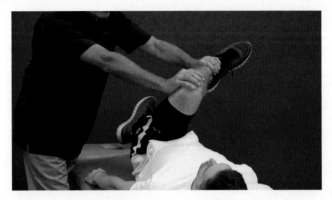

- If this maneuver reproduces the patient's pain, think IT band, trochanteric bursitis, or hip extender (hamstring, piriformis, gluteal) dysfunction.

Palpation

- Palpate the region of discomfort to try to reproduce symptoms.
- If not severely tender, perform stretch/relax treatment on the involved muscle groups.
- If severely tender, perform reciprocal inhibition (shown below, pages 159-161).

Remember the Rules

1. Move to a position of less pain and apply trigger point care.
2. Stretch the SHORTENED muscle.
3. Treat the region (above and below pain).
4. Tape to support neutral position.
5. Support definitive treatment (physical therapy, orthopedics, neurosurgery).

Treatments

If pain is not severe:

Posterior Leg Pain (Hamstrings, Piriformis, Gluteals)

- With the patient supine, lift the affected leg, keeping the knee straight until an end point is reached.
- Rest the patient's ankle on your shoulder. With the other hand, grasp the thigh just proximal to the knee. If the discomfort is too great, this movement can be performed with the knee slightly bent.
- Instruct the patient to try to lower their leg toward the table against your shoulder, using 10% effort for three belly breaths.

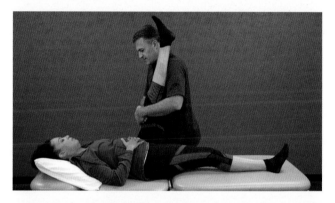

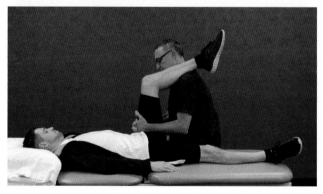

- Have the patient relax and move the hip into further flexion.
- Repeat this cycle for a total of three contract-relax cycles.

Piriformis (Tight Hip Extensor Sometimes Causing Sciatica)

Supine

- Have the patient flex their hip and knee on the involved side.
- Place your hands on the patient's knee and ankle and move the knee toward the opposite shoulder to the end point.
- Have the patient use 10% effort to try to externally rotate the leg by moving both the knee and the ankle against you while taking three belly breaths.
- Have the patient relax while you move the knee further toward the opposite shoulder.
- Repeat these steps for a total of three stretch-relax cycles.

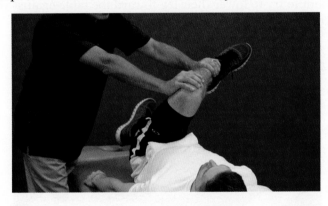

Prone

- To perform this treatment with the patient prone:
- Have the patient put the feet together and flex the involved knee.
- Move the involved ankle externally (internal rotation of the thigh) until it reaches an end point.
- Provide resistance while you instruct the patient to use 10% effort to move the ankle to the midline against your hand and take three belly breaths.
- Have the patient relax while you move the ankle further away from the midline.
- Follow these steps for three stretch-relax cycles.
- A soft tissue release can also be done here by applying pressure to the piriformis region with your fist while moving the patient's ankle and hip into external and internal rotation.

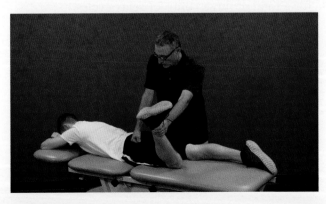

ⓘ Reciprocal Inhibition When Severe Pain Is Present for Posterior Leg Pain

If the above-mentioned stretches are too painful, perform reciprocal inhibition.

- With the patient supine, flex the hip until it reaches the end point, then back off slightly, and cross your hands over the patient's anterior thigh.
- Ask the patient to lift their leg toward their head with 10% effort against resistance, while taking three belly breaths.

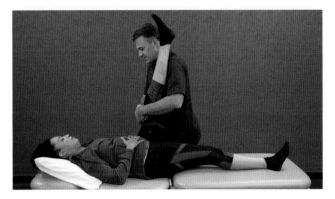

- Have the patient relax and move to a new limit.
- Repeat these steps for three cycles.

Hip Flexor Stretches for Anterior Hip Pain

Supine

- With the patient supine, place the involved leg off the end of the table.
- Flex the patient's other hip and knee.
- Hold both knees stable and ask the patient to raise the involved knee against your resistance while taking three belly breaths, then relax; move the involved leg further into a stretch.
- Repeat these steps for three stretch-relax cycles.

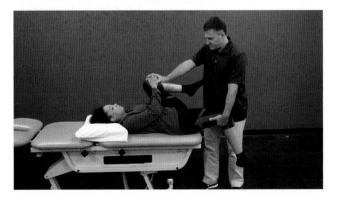

Prone (use if patient more comfortable in prone)

- With the patient prone and involved knee flexed, lift the involved leg off the table to the end point while stablizing the ipsalateral **PSIS** with your other hand.
- Ask the patient to gently bring the knee down toward the table, using 10% effort, against resistance for three belly breaths.
- Have the patient relax and move the hip further into extension.
- Repeat these steps for total of three cycles.

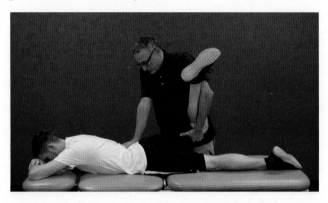

⊙ Reciprocal Inhibition for Hip Flexor Tightness

- With the patient's involved leg hanging off the end of the table and the opposite knee and hip flexed, place one hand on the uninvolved knee and gently flex the involved thigh to the end point with the other hand.

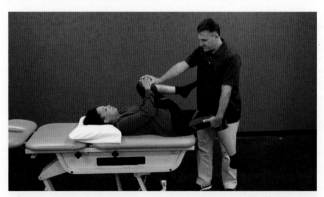

- Ask the patient to use 10% effort to try to bring the thigh down against resistance while taking three belly breaths.
- Then ask the patient to relax while you move the involved leg further into hip extension to the end point (you can also add more hip flexion on the opposite side if it makes the patient feel better.)
- Repeat these steps for three stretch-relax cycles.

ILIOTIBIAL BAND DYSFUNCTION

If the patient has lateral hip pain or pain over the lateral aspect of the proximal tibia, the IT band may be the cause. Two tests can be attempted to diagnose IT band dysfunction, the Noble Compression Test and the Ober Test. First attempt the Noble, then Ober; if the patient has positive findings, you can treat the IT Band from the Ober testing position.

Diagnosis
Noble Compression Test

- With the patient supine, flex the knee and hip to 90 degrees.
- Apply pressure with your thumb 1 to 2 cm proximal to the lateral femoral condyle.
- While maintaining this pressure, have the patient slowly extend the knee; if this induces pain either at the hip or over the lateral aspect of the proximal tibia, they likely have IT band dysfunction.

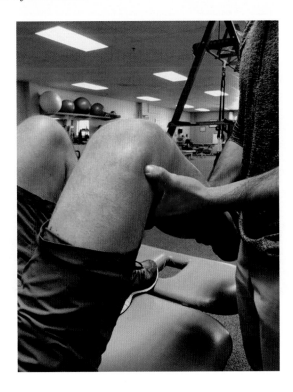

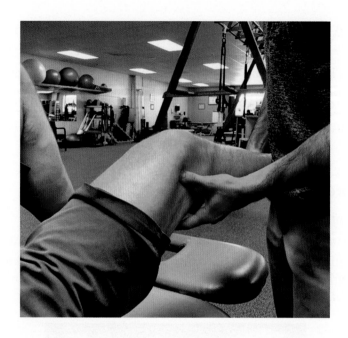

▶ Ober Test

- Assist the patient into a side-lying position with the uninvolved side down and the lower hip and knee flexed.

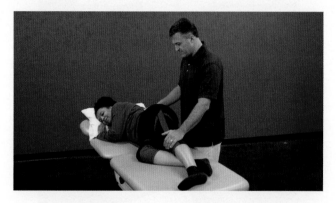

- Move the involved hip into extension and allow it to fall toward the floor, while maintaining contact with the anterior superior iliac spine.

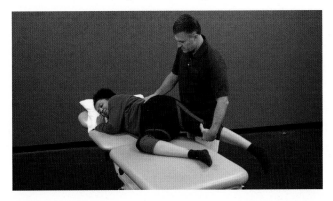

- If the patient has pain or the leg has decreased range of motion, this test is positive for IT band restriction.

Treatment
▶ Hold/Relax for Iliotibial Band

- From the Ober test position, move the patient's leg to fall toward the floor as far as possible, keeping the pelvis perpendicular to the table.
- Ensure a neutral lumbar spine.
- Place one hand on the hip and the other on the knee, and hold resistance while the patient, using 10% effort, tries to lift the ankle and knee vertically for three belly breaths.

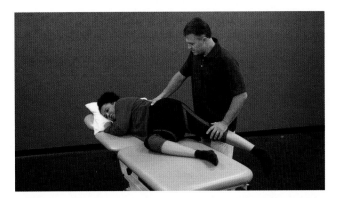

- Have the patient relax while you move the leg into further adduction.
- Repeat these steps for a total of three stretch-relax cycles.
- If performing the Ober test causes a great deal of discomfort, attempt "Adductor Stretch via Reciprocal Inhibition of the Iliotibial Band" (see page 164).

ADDUCTOR DYSFUNCTION

Treatment

⊙ Adductor Stretch and Reciprocal Inhibition of Iliotibial Band

- If testing for IT band dysfunction causes severe pain and the adductors are tight, perform reciprocal inhibition of the IT band.
- If the patient has tight adductor muscles on FABER testing, use this adductor stretch.
- With the patient supine, move the involved leg laterally off the table to an end point supporting the medial aspect of the knee and lower leg.

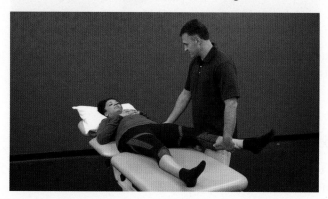

- Ask the patient to try to move the leg back toward the midline, keeping the opposite pelvis stationary, for three belly breaths.
- Have the patient relax and move the leg further into abduction laterally.
- Repeat these steps for a total of three stretch-relax cycles.

⊙ External Rotation Adductor Stretch

- With the patient supine, move the involved side to the edge of the table and have the patient flex the hip and externally rotate the leg to an end point, placing the foot against your hip.
- Place one hand on the opposite ASIS/hip and the other on the involved knee.

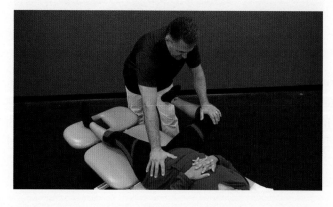

- Ask the patient to use 10% effort to push into your hip while trying to internally rotate the hip for three belly breaths.
- Have the patient relax while you move the hip further into external rotation.
- Repeat these steps for a total of three stretch-relax cycles.

Treatment Summary

Posterior Leg Pain

1.

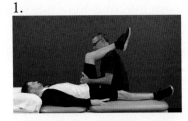

Piriformis

1.

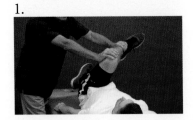

2.

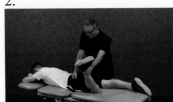

Reciprocal Inhibition When Severe Pain is Present for Posterior Leg Pain

1.

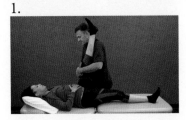

Hip Flexor Stretches for Anterior Thigh Pain

1.

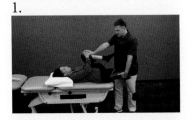

2.

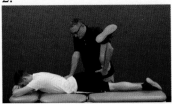

Reciprocal Inhibition for Hip Flexor Tightness

1.

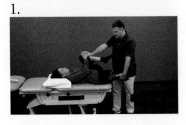

Hold/Relax for Iliotibial Band

1.

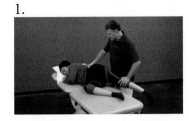

Reciprocal Inhibition of Iliotibial Band via Adductor Stretch.

1.

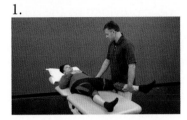

External Rotation Adductor Stretch

1.

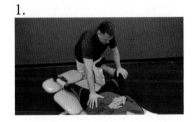

Sample Procedure Notes and Coding

Procedure:	CPT Codes 99140 x X units ICD-10-CM Diagnosis Code(s): 99213 or 99214 Hip Pain, Unspecified M25.559 Strain, Right Hip S76.011 Strain, Left Hip S76.012S99070 – Supplies and Materials: provided by the qualified health care professional over and above those usually included with the office visit (list supplies/materials used)
Informed consent	After explaining the risks, benefits, and alternatives for the treatment, the patient gave verbal consent for the procedure
Description of Procedure	
Outcomes/Complications	__none; other:
Instructions to Patient	
Time	Total time spent in **constant attendance** with the patient performing manual therapies: XX minutes

For all hip and upper leg pain, perform the self FABER stretch first.

Perform both self FABER exercises; if one hurts, just do the other.

- Lie on your back and cross your leg over your opposite knee.

- Using your hands, gently push your knee away from your head while taking three belly breaths.

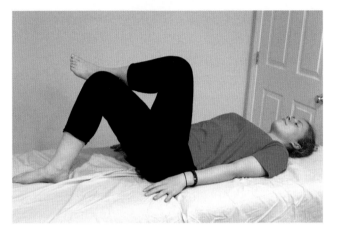

- Then gently PULL your knee toward the OPPOSITE shoulder while taking three belly breaths.

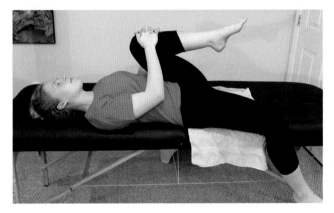

- If either motion hurts, do not repeat. Repeat the motion that produces most improvement, and do both if both improve symptoms.

Lying Hip Stretch

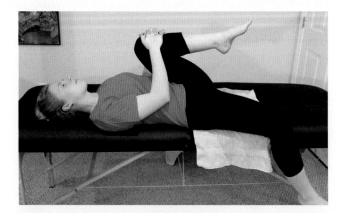

- Allow the involved leg to hang over side of table, and bring the opposite knee up toward your chest.
- Take three belly breaths and try to allow muscles holding the involved leg to relax. You may even use 1- to 5-lb ankle weight to stretch further.

Bridges

- Flex your hips and knees to about 45 degrees.

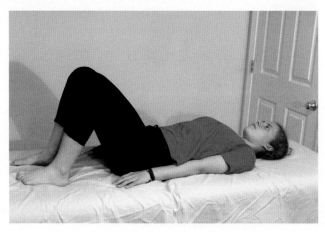

- Push your feet down, lifting you buttocks and back off the bed.

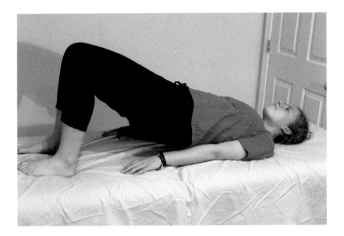

- Hold for three belly breaths, then relax.

Perform the self FABER stretches first, then perform this exercise.

Standing Hamstring Stretch

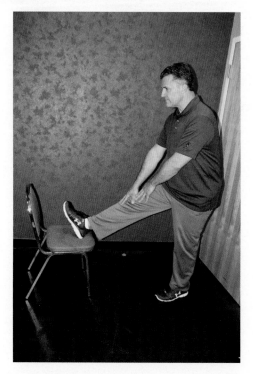

- Place the involved leg on a table, sofa arm rest, or—if those options are too painful—a chair.
- Keeping your back straight, gently push your heel down while taking three belly breaths, then relax.
- Repeat these steps three times.

Perform the self FABER stretches first, then perform this exercise.

• Place the involved ankle over the opposite knee.

• Press down gently on the involved knee while taking three belly breaths, then relax.

• Repeat these steps three times.

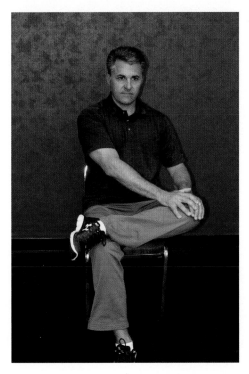

Perform the self FABER stretches first, then perform this exercise.
- Sit with involved leg crossed over other knee.

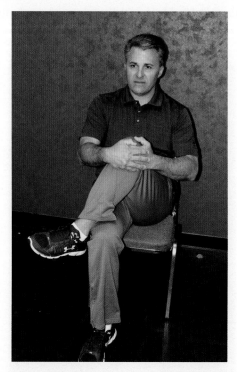

- Pull the knee toward the opposite shoulder, and take three belly breaths and relax.
- Repeat for three stretch-relax cycles.

Perform the self FABER stretches first, then perform this exercise.

Side-Lying: Iliotibial Band Stretch

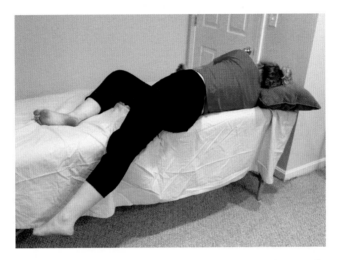

- Lie with the involved leg up and bend the uninvolved knee forward.
- Allow your involved leg, with your knee straight, to hang over the side of table.
- Take three belly breaths and relax.
- You may put a 1- to 5-lb weight on ankle to help further stretch the IT band.

Figure Credits

Iliac Crest Height: Reprinted from Callaghan JJ, Rosenberg AG, Rubash HE, et al. The Adult Hip. Philadelphia: Wolters Kluwer; 2015 with permission.

Bridges: Reprinted from Williams A. Study Guide to Accompany Massage Mastery: Theory and Technique. Baltimore: Wolters Kluwer; 2012 with permission.

CHAPTER | 12
KNEE PAIN

Introduction

Knee pain can occur from direct injury to its bone, meniscus, and ligaments or can be referred from more proximal muscles and hip (Figure 12-1).

Differential Diagnosis

The differential diagnosis for knee pain includes tight hamstrings, tight quadriceps, iliotibial (IT) band syndrome, anserine bursitis, meniscal injury, anterior cruciate ligament (ACL) injury, and patellar tendon dysfunction. Conditions that are amenable to manual medicine include patellofemoral syndrome, patellar tendonitis, IT band dysfunction, and anserine bursitis with adductor dysfunction.

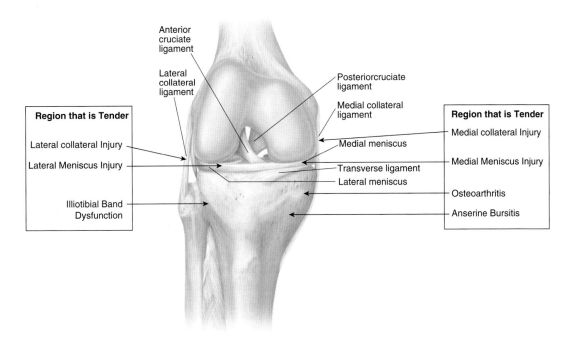

Figure 12-1 • Locations of common injuries and dysfunctions of the knee.

Acute Knee Pain

- History of trauma or new activities
- Differential diagnosis includes disruption of the ACL, posterior cruciate ligament (PCL), lateral or medial collateral ligaments or meniscal injuries

Diagnosis

- **Acute pain without trauma**
  - Common causes: osteoarthritis, infectious (Lyme, gonorrhea), gout
- **General knee pain with swelling** (loss of prepatellar medial and/or lateral concavities) (Figure 12-2)
  - If the knee swells within 2 hours after new activity, think ACL injury.
  - If the knee swells a few hours after a new activity, think meniscal or colateral ligament injury.
- **Generalized knee pain with little or no edema**
  - Common causes: patella-femoral pain, patellar tendonitis, derangement from within the joint (from meniscal injury or cyst)
- **Lateral knee pain**
  - Common causes: lateral collateral injury, IT band dysfunction, lateral meniscus injury
  - Pain over the lateral joint line: lateral collateral sprain or tear
  - Pain on palpation over the anterolateral joint space: may imply lateral meniscus injury
  - Pain over proximal tibia laterally: test for IT band dysfunction.

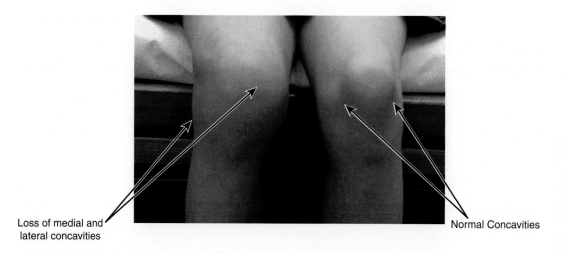

Loss of medial and lateral concavities

Normal Concavities

Figure 12-2 • Normal versus lost concavities. (Reprinted from Fisher RG, Boyce TH, Correa AG. *Moffet's Pediatric Infectious Diseases*. Philadelphia: Wolters Kluwer; 2017 with permission.)

- **Medial knee pain**
  - Common causes: medial collateral injury, osteoarthritis, medial meniscus injury, anserine bursitis.
  - Pain on palpation over the medial joint line: medial collateral sprain or tear or osteoarthritis
  - Pain on palpation anteriorly over proximal tibia: could be due to anserine bursitis or osteoarthritis
  - Pain on palpation over anteromedial joint line: medial meniscal injury
- Treatment for suspected collateral ligament injury or partial tear, ACL/PCL injury, or meniscal injury, treat with RISE (**R**est, **I**ce, **C**ompression, **E**levation) and refer to physical therapy for rehabilitation treatment.
- X-rays are indicated if fracture is suspected. Magnetic resonance imaging is rarely initially necessary unless patient fails physical therapy.

Remember the Rules

1. Move to a position of less pain and apply trigger point care.
2. Stretch the SHORTENED muscle.
3. Treat the region (above and below pain).
4. Tape to support neutral position.
5. Support definitive treatment (physical therapy, orthopedics, neurosurgery).

GENERALIZED KNEE PAIN

Diagnosis

Patellofemoral Syndrome

- Proximal/generalized patellar pain, often due to quadriceps dysfunction with tight IT band and weak vastus medialis oblique (VMO): patella track *laterally* and compresses into the lateral femoral condyle.
- Perform patellar compression test
  - Position the patient supine and relaxed.
  - Push posteriorly on patella, and ask patient to contract the quadriceps.
  - If pain is elicited, patellofemoral syndrome is likely.

Patellar Tendonitis/Jumper Knee

- Distal patellar pain due to distal patellar tendon inflammation, often related to tight hamstring and quadriceps, overuse, or faulty foot mechanics.
- Patellar Tendonitis Test
  - Position the patient supine and relaxed.
  - Press down on the proximal aspect of the patella with your superior thumb.
  - Using the other hand, push under the inferior pole of the patella.
  - If pain occurs at the distal aspect, think patellar tendonitis.

Treatment for Patellofemoral Syndrome and Patellar Tendonitis

Treatment involves addressing tight quadriceps.

Hip Flexor Stretches

Supine

- With the patient supine, place the involved leg off the end of the table.
- Flex the patient's other hip and knee.
- Hold both knees stable, and ask the patient to raise the involved knee against your resistance while taking three belly breathes, then relax; move the involved leg further into an extension stretch.
- Repeat these steps for three stretch-relax cycles.

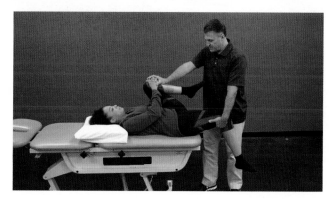

Prone

- With the patient prone and involved knee flexed, lift the involved leg off the table to the end point.
- Ask the patient to gently bring the knee down toward the table, using 10% effort, against resistance for three belly breaths.
- Have the patient relax and move the hip further into extension.
- Repeat these steps for total of three cycles.

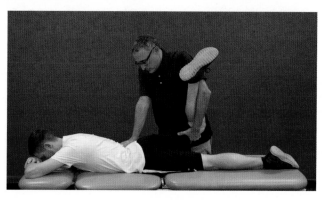

- If this stretch is too painful, perform reciprocal inhibition.

⊙ Reciprocal Inhibition for Hip Flexor Tightness

- With the patient supine and the involved leg hanging off the end of the table and the opposite knee and hip flexed, place one hand on the uninvolved knee and gently lift the involved thigh to the end point with the other hand.

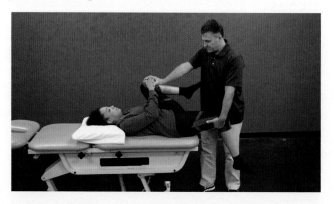

- Ask the patient to use 10% effort to try to bring the thigh down against resistance while taking three belly breaths.
- Then ask the patient to relax while you move the involved leg further into hip extension to the end point (you can also add more hip flexion on the opposite side, if it makes the patient feel better.)
- Repeat these steps for three stretch-relax cycles.

⊙ Kinesiology Taping for Patellar Tendonitis

- Have the patient sitting with the knee flexed off the end of the table.
- Measure the strip from the mid-thigh to the distal aspect of the patellar tendon, then double the length of the tape and cut.
- Cut a second 6-inch strip.
- Split the long piece of tape in the middle and stretch it 50% tension. Apply over the infra-patellar tendon.

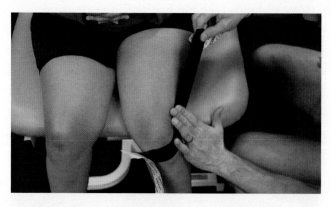

- Maintain 50% tension as you apply each side proximally up the medial and lateral thigh. Apply the last 2 inches on each side without tension. Rub the tape to activate the adhesive.

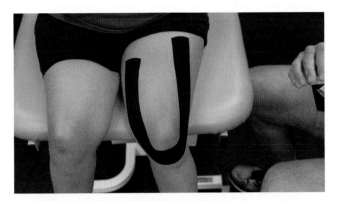

- Split the middle of the second piece of tape and apply across the inferior patellar tendon, applying the last 2 inch without tension.

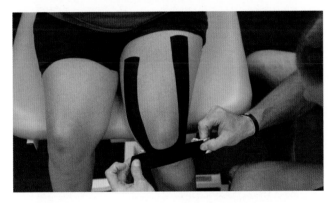

- Rub to activate the adhesive.

ILIOTIBIAL BAND FRICTION SYNDROME CAUSING LATERAL KNEE PAIN

Figure 12-3 shows the anatomy of the IT band.

Diagnosis

- Testing the IT Band can be done using the Noble Compression Test or the Ober Test.

Noble Compression Test

- With the patient supine, flex the knee and hip to 90 degrees.
- Apply pressure with your thumb 1 to 2 cm proximal to the lateral femoral condyle.

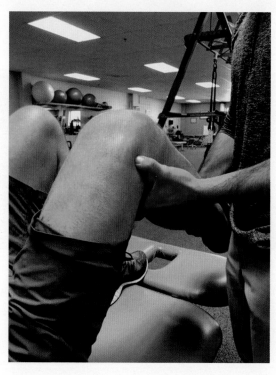

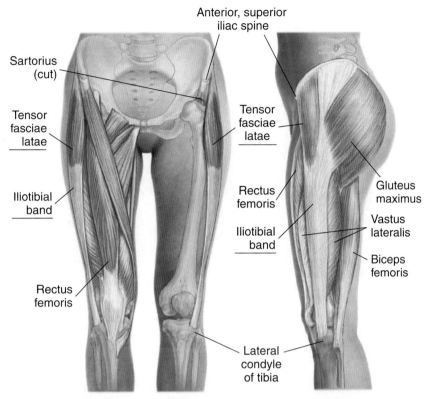

Figure 12-3 • Anatomy of the tensor fasciae latae and the iliotibial band. (Reprinted from Clay JH, Allen L, Pounds DM. *Clay and Pound's Basic Clinical Massage Therapy*. Baltimore: Wolters Kluwer; 2015 with permission.)

• While maintaining this pressure, have the patient slowly extend the knee; if this induces their pain, they likely have IT band dysfunction.

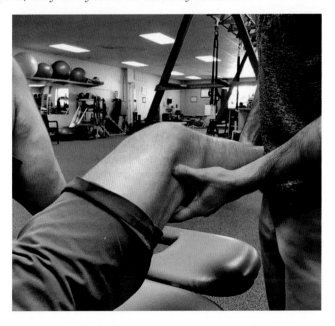

▶ Ober Test

- Next, assist the patient into a side-lying position. Ask the patient to move toward the side of the table closest to you with the uninvolved side down and the lower hip and knee flexed.

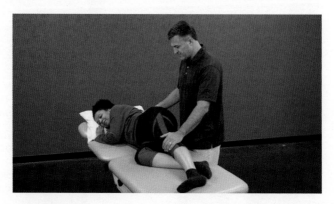

- Move the involved hip into extension, and allow it to fall toward the floor, while maintaining contact with the anterior superior iliac spine.
- If the patient has pain or the leg has decreased range of motion as it moves towards the floor, the test is positive for IT band restriction.

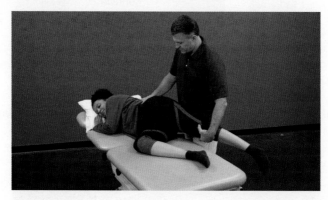

Treatment for Iliotibial Band Syndrome

▶ Hold/Relax for Iliotibial Band

- From the Ober test position, allow the patient's leg to fall toward the floor as far as possible, keeping the pelvis perpendicular to the table.
- Ensure a neutral lumbar spine.
- Place one hand on the hip and the other on the knee, and hold resistance while the patient, using 10% effort, tries to lift the ankle and knee vertically for three belly breaths.

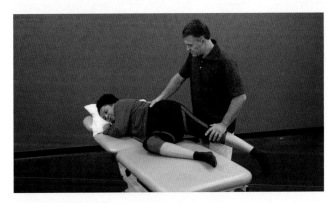

- Have the patient relax while you move the leg into further adduction.
- Repeat these steps for total of three cycles.

▶ Kinesiology Taping for Iliotibial Band Friction Syndrome

- Have the patient lie with the involved side up.
- Measure a strip from the patient's hip to just distal to the knee joint line.
- Cut a second strip to about 6 inches.
- Attach the first 2 inches of tape at the top of the ilium without tension.
- Using 25% to 50% stretch, apply the tape down the lateral aspect of the thigh to just below the knee to the proximal lateral tibial tubercle.

- Apply the last 2 inch without tension.
- Rub the tape to activate the adhesive.

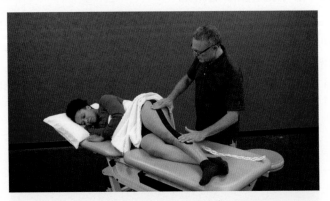

- Tear the paper in center of the smaller strip and apply a 50% stretch.
- Place perpendicular to the long strip, just proximal to the knee joint.

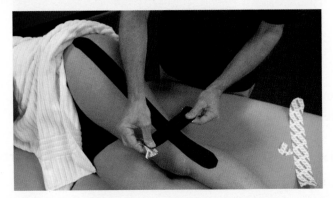

- Rub the tape to activate the adhesive.

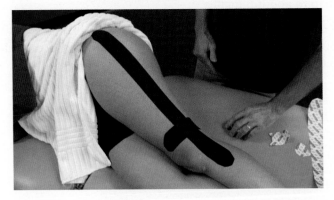

ANSERINE BURSITIS AND HIP ADDUCTOR DYSFUNCTION CAUSING MEDIAL KNEE PAIN

Diagnosis

- Symptoms of medial knee pain, typically after starting new activity

Examination

- Point tenderness over anserine bursa without joint line tenderness (Figure 12-4)

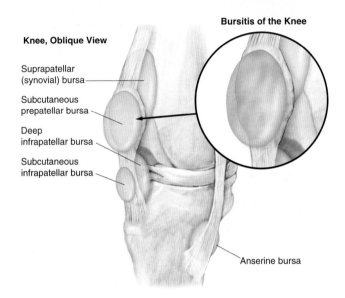

Figure 12-4 • Right knee, medial oblique view showing the bursae. (Reprinted from Anatomical Chart Company with permission from Wolters Kluwer.)

Treatment

- With the patient supine, move the involved leg into abduction to its end point, keeping the toes pointing toward the ceiling.
- Hold the calcaneus and use your forearm to prevent the toes from turning out.
- Using the other hand, roll the opposite hip and knee away (external hip rotation) while keeping the involved hip down on the table.
- Move your hip against the medial aspect of the patient's ankle and ask the patient to adduct/push into your hip, using 10% effort, while holding resistance for five counts.

- Have the patient relax and take three belly breaths while you move the leg further into abduction to a new end point.
- Repeat these steps for total of three cycles.

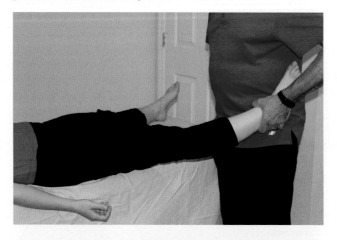

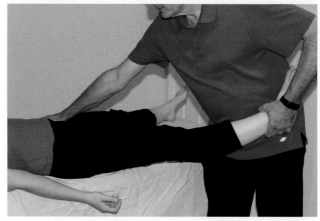

⊙ External Rotation Adductor Stretch

- With the patient supine, move the involved side to the edge of the table and have the patient flex the hip and externally rotate the leg to an end point, placing the foot against your hip.
- Place one hand on the opposite anterior superior iliac spine (ASIS)/hip and the other on the involved knee.

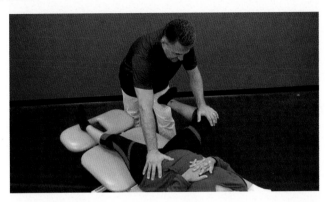

- Ask the patient to use 10% effort to internally rotate the hip for three belly breaths.
- Have the patient relax while you move the hip further into external rotation.
- Repeat these steps for a total of three stretch-relax cycles.

⊙ Kinesiology Taping for Anserine Bursitis

- Have the patient sit at the end of the table with the leg hanging off the edge. Cut two pieces of tape 6 to 8 inches in length.
- Attach the first 2 inches of tape without tension above the knee so that the tape hangs at an angle toward the medial malleolus.
- Pull with a 50% stretch across the medial joint line and attach the tape to the proximal tibia.

- Attach the last 2 inches with no stretch.
- Rub the tape to activate the adhesive.

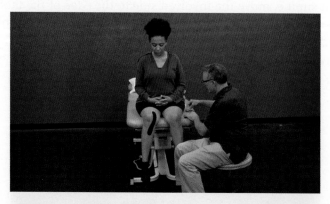

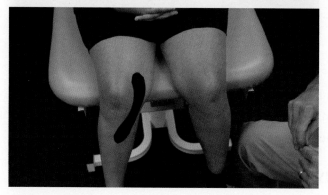

- Apply the second strip, medial to the first piece of tape, with the initial 2 inches without tension. Then, with a 50% stretch, apply over the anserine bursa and under that patella.
- Attach the last 2 inches with no tension.

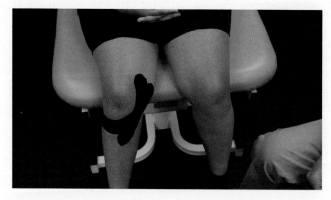

- Rub the tape to activate the adhesive.

Treatment Summary

Treatment for Patellofemoral Syndrome and Patellar Tendonitis

Hip Flexor Stretches

1.
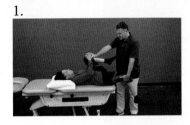

2.
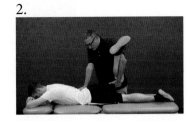

Reciprocal Inhibition for Hip Flexor Tightness

1.
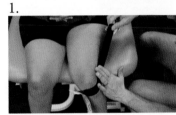

Kinesiology Taping for Patellar Tendonitis

1.
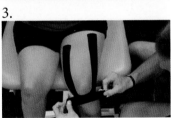

2.
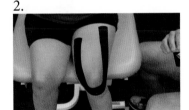

3.
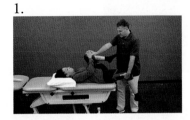

Iliotibial Band Friction Syndrome Causing Lateral Knee Pain

Hold/Relax for Iliotibial Band

1.

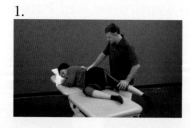

Kinesiology Taping for Iliotibial Band Friction Syndrome

1.

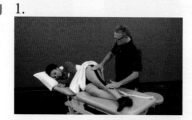

2.

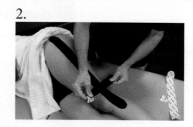

3.

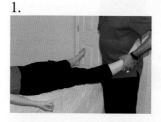

Anserine Bursitis and Hip Adductor Dysfunction Causing Medial Knee Pain

Adductor Stretch

1.

2.

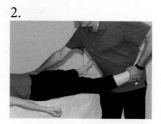

External Rotation Adductor Stretch

1.

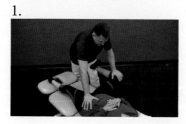

1.

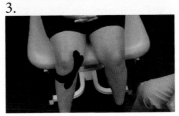

2.

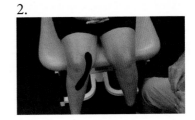

3.

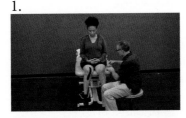

Sample Procedure Notes and Coding

Procedure:	**ICD-10-CM Diagnosis Codes:**
	Patellofemoral Disorders: M22.2X9 Patellar Tendonitis: **M76.50** Iliotibial Band Dysfunction: **M76.30** Anserine Bursitis: M70.50 Adductor Dysfunction: S76.219S **CPT**: 97140 – Manual therapy techniques one or more regions

Minutes	Units Reported
8-22	1
23-37	2
38-52	3
53-67	4

	99070 – Supplies and Materials: provided by the qualified health care professional over and above those usually included with the office visit (list supplies/materials used)
Informed Consent	After explaining the risks, benefits, and alternatives for the treatment, the patient gave verbal consent for the procedure
Description of Procedure	
Outcomes/ Complications	
Instructions to Patient	
Time	Total time spent in **constant attendance** with the patient performing manual therapies: XX minutes

Hamstring Bridge

- Lie on your back with your knees bent and your feet resting on the floor.
- Keep your knees and feet hip width apart and your toes facing forward with your ankles below your knees.
- Stretch your arms straight beside your body with palms facing downward.
- Squeeze your hamstrings and your buttocks, press down through your heels and lift your hips off the mat.
- Hold the bridge position for 10 to 20 seconds, then lower your hips back to the floor.
- Repeat these steps 10 to 15 times, two to three times a day.

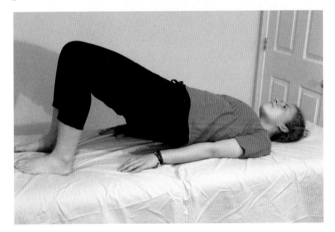

Glute Bridge

- Lie on your back with the knees bent so the feet are flat on the table and ankles are below your knees.
- Place your hands at your side with palms facing downward.
- Lift your toes so only heels are on the table.
- Tighten your abdomen and squeeze your glutes while pushing downward through your heels to lift hips up off table.

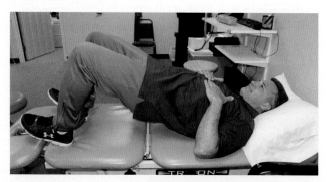

- To increase the challenge, cross your arms in front of your chest while performing this glute bridge.
- Hold this position for 10 to 20 seconds, then lower your hips back to the floor.
- Repeat these steps 10 to 15 times, two to three times/day.

Quadriceps Stretch

- Place a belt or stretching strap around your ankle and lie on your stomach.
- Slowly bend your affected knee as far as you can, pulling the belt with your hands (as shown) until a gentle stretch is felt over the front of your thigh, the quadriceps muscles.

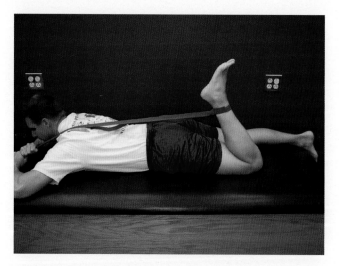

- Hold this position for 20 to 30 seconds.
- Repeat these steps 10-15 times, two to three times a day.

Quad Sets

- Lie with your leg as straight as possible.

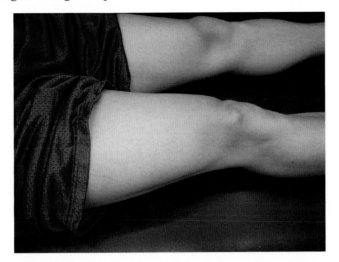

- Gently push your knee into the floor or surface you are lying on by tightening your thigh muscle.

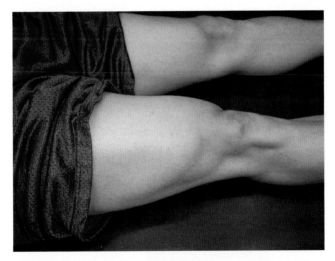

- If this is too hard, roll a towel and place behind your knee.
- If the quadriceps muscles do not seem to tighten, gently tap on them to help your body relearn to contract them.
- Hold the contraction for 8 to 10 seconds.
- Repeat these steps for three sets of 10 contractions.

Hamstring Stretch

- Lie on your back with your knee straight and your hand supporting the leg behind knee.
- Slowly pull the back of the knee until a stretch is felt in the back of the thigh.

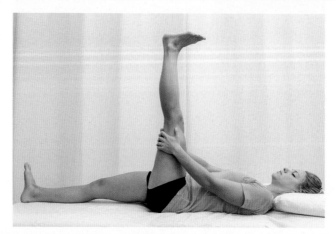

- Hold this position for 20 to 30 seconds.
- Repeat these steps three to five times, for two to three sets/day.

Adductor Dysfunction

- Lie on your back and cross your leg over your opposite knee. Stay in this position if a stretch is felt.
- When a stretch is no longer felt, gently push the knee away from you with your hands and hold 20 to 30 seconds.

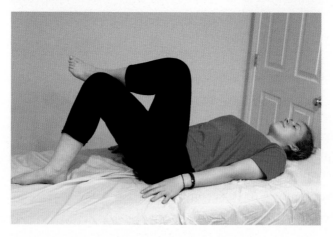

- Repeat these steps three to five times for one to two sets.

Selected References

Kaya M, ErcinE, Razak Ozdıncler A, Ones N. A comparison of two manual physical therapy approaches and electrotherapy modalities for patients with knee osteoarthritis: a randomized three arm clinical trial. *Physiother Theor Pract*. 2018;34(8):600-612. doi:10.1080/09593985.2018.14 23591. Epub 2018 Jan 8.

Weckström K, Söderström J. Radial extracorporeal shockwave therapy compared with manual therapy in runners with iliotibial band syndrome. *J Back Musculoskelet Rehabil*. 2016;29(1):161-170. doi:10.3233/BMR-150612.

Figure Credits

Hamstring stretch: Reprinted from Donnelly JM, Fernández-de-Las-Peñas C, Finnegan M, Freeman JL. *Travell, Simons & Simons' Myofascial Pain and Dysfunction*. Philadelphia: Wolters Kluwer; 2018 with permission.

Quad sets and quadriceps stretch: Reprinted from Lotke OA, Abboud JA, Ende J. *Lippincott"s Primary Care Orthopaedics*. Philadelphia: Wolters Kluwer; 2013 with permission.

CHAPTER | 13
FOOT AND ANKLE PAIN

Introduction

When approaching foot and ankle complaints, first be certain to rule out missed fractures or incomplete rehabilitation of a previous ankle sprain.

Common causes of ankle pain include plantar fasciitis, acute and chronic ankle sprain, chronic lateral ankle pain (due to tendonitis and/or incomplete rehabilitation of an old ankle sprain), Achilles tendonitis, lateral ankle pain due to peroneal tendonitis, medial ankle pain due to shin splints and posterior tibial tendonitis (also called tarsal tunnel syndrome), bunions, and gout. Uncommon causes include missed medial or lateral malleolus fracture, unhealed fifth metatarsal fractures, and navicular fractures.

PLANTAR FASCIITIS

Diagnosis

- Pain on plantar surface, usually at the calcaneal insertion of plantar fascia, pain increased upon initial weight bearing, especially in the morning or on initiation of walking after prolonged rest.
- Due to degenerative change of plantar fascia at origin on medial tuberosity of calcaneus, and related to obesity, flat feet (pes planus), tight heel cord, and/or lack of mobility of tibialis anterior and in the lower leg from fascial adhesion.

Treatment
⊙ Soft Tissue Mobilization of Plantar Fascia

- Move the patient's foot into inversion and palpate along the plantar fascia for tender points.

- While holding pressure on the tender point, move the foot into eversion.

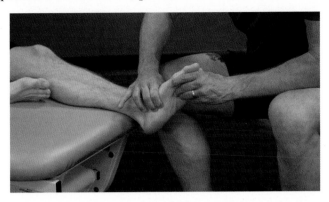

- Move further distally along the fascia and repeat.

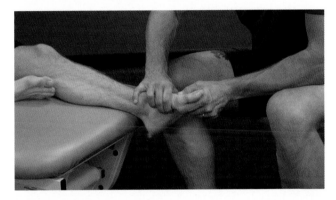

▶ Tibialis Anterior Mobilization

- Palpate just lateral to the tibia (along tibialis anterior) for tender points.
- Using your hand or a ball, hold the tender point in place, and ask the patient to plantar flex and dorsiflex the foot 10 times.
- Repeat this process just medial to the tibia.
- If this movement causes any distal paresthesias, apply less pressure before continuing.

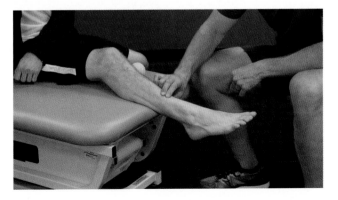

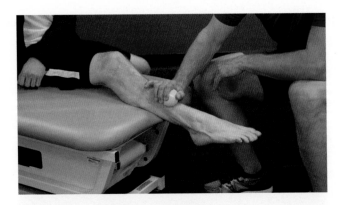

▶ Active Release for Plantar Fasciitis

- The patient sits with the leg straight.

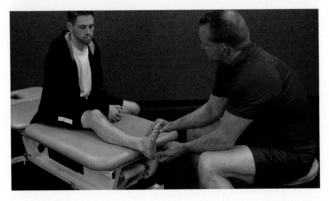

- While you apply pressure to the tender spots on the distal calcaneus and plantar fascia, ask the patient to bend the toes down, or plantar flex the toes, while keeping the knee flat on the table.

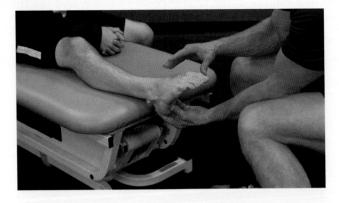

- Hold the toes in resistance while asking the patient to dorsiflex the toes, then relax.
- Move gradually along the plantar fascia repeating the process of toe plantar flexion, holding pressure on the tender spots, then dorsiflexion against resistance.

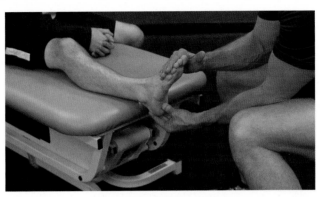

▶ Navicular Sling for Plantar Fasciitis

- Have the patient keep the foot and ankle relaxed.
- Anchor athletic tape just inferior to the lateral malleolus, then apply it to the plantar aspect of the foot along the calcaneus.

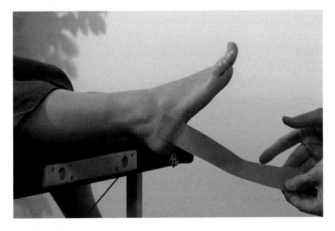

- While grasping the calcaneus, move the foot into inversion as far as you can without causing pain, and pull with the tape, moving the foot into further inversion.
- Attach the tape over the medial aspect of the foot and then across the anterior aspect of the mid foot.

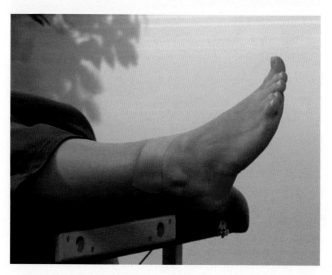

- Repeat the process with a second length of tape covering the first piece of tape, again by inverting the foot and pulling the foot into inversion with the tape.

Other Treatments

- Self-massage with a frozen bottle of water

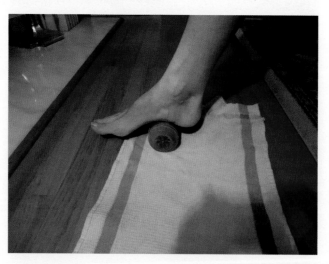

- Weight reduction if body mass index is greater than 25
- Orthotics and plantar fasciitis straps: beneficial in combination with a short course of nonsteroidal anti-inflammatory drugs (NSAIDs)
- Night splints: can be initially uncomfortable; better tolerated over time
- Foam roller or tennis ball to areas just lateral and medial to tibia

ACUTE LATERAL ANKLE SPRAIN

Diagnosis

- Inversion injury of the ankle is the most common ankle sprain, involving the anterior talofibular ligaments. X-rays are not needed unless it meets the requirements of the Ottawa Rules.
- Ottawa Rules. For those aged 18 to 50 years, an ankle x-ray series is required only if there is:
  - Bone tenderness at the posterior edge or tip of the lateral malleolus

    or
  - Bone tenderness at the posterior edge or tip of the medial malleolus

    or
  - Bone tenderness at the base of the fifth metatarsal

    or
  - Bone tenderness at the navicular

    or
  - An inability to bear weight both immediately after the injury and in the emergency department for four steps (Figure 13-1)

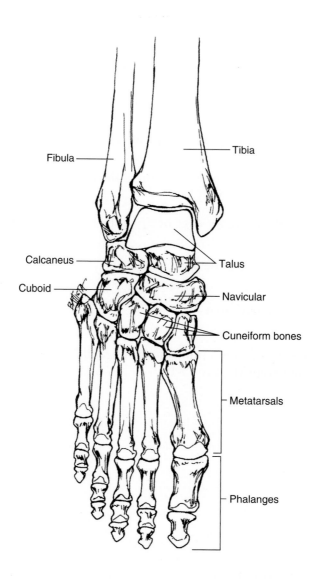

Figure 13-1 • Typical fracture locations include the medial and lateral malleolus, the navicular, and the base of the fifth metatarsal. (Reprinted from Oatis CA. *Kinesiology*. 2nd ed. Baltimore: Wolters Kluwer; 2016 with permission.)

Treatment

▶ Spiral Tape for Acute Inversion Sprain

- Cut a strip of athletic tape 1½ times around the ankle.
- Place the foot in a neutral position.
- Apply the tape starting anterior to and just superior to the lateral malleolus, having the malleolus visible inferior to the tape.

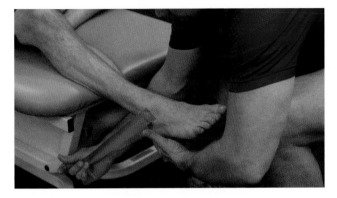

- Mobilize the distal fibula posteriorly and up with your thumb.
- Pull the tape superiorly at 45-degree angle, then posteriorly up and around the ankle and secure it to the anterior leg just above the ankle, but do not let the tape contact the beginning end.

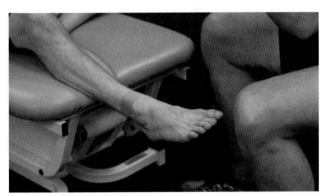

- Rub the tape to help the adhesive attach.
- Apply a second piece of tape over the first, again starting at the lateral side of the ankle.
- Mobilize the distal fibula posteriorly and up, and pull on the tape while applying it again over the first piece of tape.

ACHILLES TENDONITIS

Diagnosis

- Painful inflammation of Achilles tendon (Figure 13-2) and its sheath due to chronic degenerative tendinosis and tearing

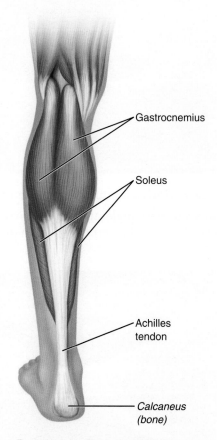

Gastrocnemius

Soleus

Achilles tendon

Calcaneus (bone)

Posterior superficial view, left leg

Figure 13-2 • Anterior and posterior view of the lower leg, including the Achilles tendon. (Reprinted from Archer PA, Nelson LA. *Applied Anatomy & Physiology for Manual Therapists*. Baltimore: Wolters Kluwer; 2012 with permission.)

Examination

- Pain and swelling along tendon with noninsertional pain and tenderness are most common.

Treatment

⏵ Calf Stretch for Achilles Tendonitis or Peroneal Tendonitis

Attempt this treatment if it is not painful.
- While prone, have the patient dorsiflex the foot on the affected side.

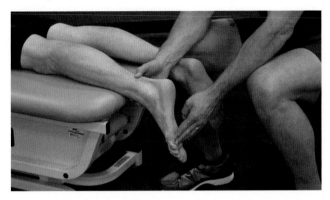

- Hold resistance over the ball of the foot while the patient tries, with 10% effort, to plantar flex the foot for three belly breathes, then relax.

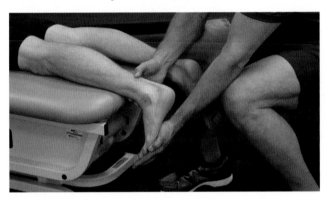

- Move the foot into further dorsiflexion and repeat these steps for a total of three stretch-relax cycles.

Trigger Point and Active Release for Achilles Tendonitis

- With the patient prone, palpate the muscles of the posterior calf for tender points.
- Hold pressure over a point and move the foot until the trigger point softens and the pain resolves.

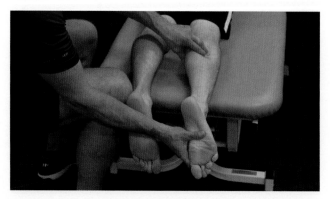

- If the trigger point starts to release, continue to hold for 90 seconds.
- If the trigger point does not release, move into an active release:
  - Hold pressure on the tender point and move the foot slowly through dorsiflexion and plantar flexion.

ⓧ Kinesiology Taping for Achilles Tendonitis

- With the patient prone, measure and cut one strip of tape from below the popliteal fossa the insertion of the Achilles tendon, and down to the distal aspect of the calcaneous the corners.
- Cut a second strip of tape about 6 to 8 inch long; round the corners.
- Starting at the base of the popliteal fossa, attach the first 2 inch of the long tape without tension.
- Using 25% to 50% stretch, apply the tape down the posterior leg and over the insertion of the Achilles tendon.
- Apply the last 2 inch without tension over the calcaneus.
- Rip the tape of the second strip in the middle, and apply it perpendicular to the long strip over the tender point of the calf.
- Rub to activate the adhesive.

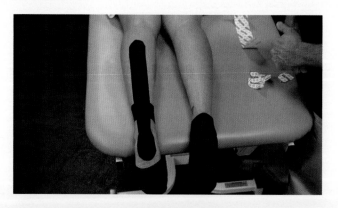

Other Treatments

- Arch support
- Foam roller to calf muscles
- Ice massage of Achilles tendon and posterior calf
- Referral to physical therapy

PERONEAL (LATERAL ANKLE) TENDONITIS

Diagnosis

- Overuse injury associated with pain over lateral ankle
- Often associated with varus knee deformity

Examination

- Tenderness is found over the lateral peroneal tendons, and weakness is found with foot eversion.
- Palpate the distal fibula (above the lateral malleolus); if tender, consider fibular stress reaction or fracture and obtain an x-ray (Figure 13-3).

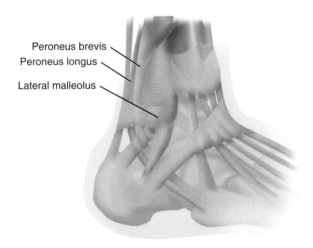

Peroneus brevis
Peroneus longus
Lateral malleolus

Figure 13-3 • Location of the distal fibula. (From Davis WH, Sobel M, Deland J, et al. The superior peroneal retinaculum: an anatomic study. *Foot Ankle Int*. 1994;15:273.)

Treatment
Calf Stretch (Attempt if Not Too Painful)

- While prone, have the patient dorsiflex the foot on the affected side.
- Hold resistance over the ball of the foot while the patient tries, with 10% effort, to plantar flex for three belly breaths, then relax.
- Move the foot into further dorsiflexion, and repeat these steps for a total of three stretch-relax cycles.

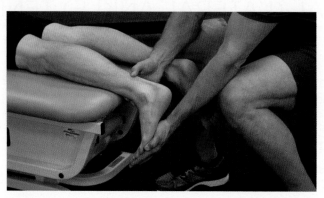

Other Treatments

- Foam roller to calf muscles
- Arch support taping—navicular sling trial
- Ice massage
- Kinesiology taping
- Referral to physical therapy

▶ Kinesiology Taping for Lateral Ankle Symptoms (Peroneal Tendonitis)

- Measure and cut a piece of tape from the medial aspect of the calcaneus to just inferior to the knee laterally
- Measure and cut a second piece of tape that will go horizontally around the calf, without overlapping.
- For the long tape, dorsiflex the foot and internally rotate.

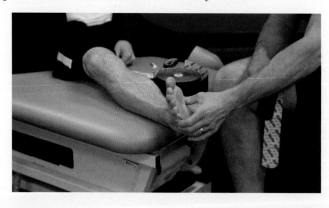

- Place 1 inch of the tape on the medial aspect of the calcaneus then tape across the calcaneus and arch; next, apply a 50% stretch and apply the tape up along the fibula region, covering the area of greatest pain.

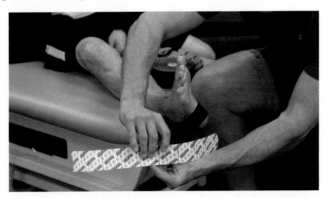

- Attach the last 3 cm with no stretch.

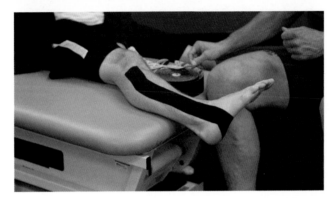

- Rub the tape to activate it.
- For the small tape, rip it in the middle.
- Stretch about 50% and apply it perpendicular to the vertical strip over the area of greatest pain.

- Secure the lateral 3 cm on each end with no stretch; then rub to activate.

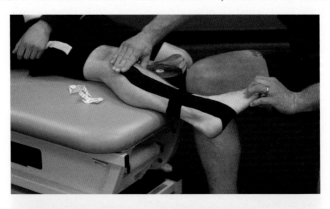

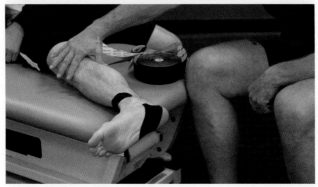

Other Treatments

- Foam roller/lateral lower leg
- Referral to physical therapy

SHIN SPLINTS (MEDIAL TIBIAL STRESS SYNDROME)

Diagnosis

- Patient reports pain over medial tibia at mid shaft with exercise; pain resolves with rest (compared with compartment syndrome, which will cause paresthesias and may lessen, but not resolve with rest, or stress fracture, which will cause pain with each heel strike that may initially resolve with rest, but ultimately causes discomfort while at rest).

Physical Examination

- Tenderness over the medial tibia at mid-shaft; also tenderness of the tibialis anterior muscle (lateral to the tibia) near the middle to distal third of the leg; pain may worsen with foot plantar flexion

Treatment

▶ Shin Splint/Anterior Tibialis Active Release

- Palpate just lateral to the tibia (along tibialis anterior) for tender points.
- Using your hand or a ball, hold the tender point in place, and ask the patient to slowly plantar flex and dorsiflex the foot 10 times.
- Repeat this process just medial to the tibia.
- If this movement causes any distal paresthesias, apply less pressure before continuing.

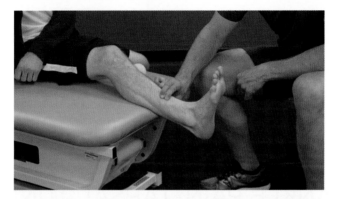

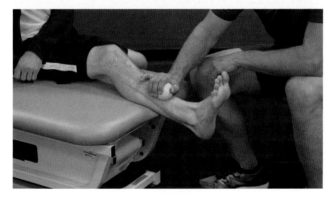

▶ Shin Splint Anterior Tibialis Stretch/Relax

- Move the foot into plantar flexion to its limit.
- Hold resistance and ask the patient to dorsiflex their foot, using 10% effort while taking three belly breaths, then relax.

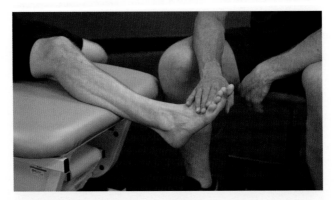

- Take up the slack and repeat these steps for a total of three stretch-relax cycles.

Kinesiology tape for shin splints (see under "Medial Ankle Pain/Tarsal Tunnel Syndrome").

MEDIAL ANKLE PAIN/TARSAL TUNNEL SYNDROME

Diagnosis

- Tarsal tunnel syndrome results from a compression neuropathy of the posterior tibial nerve as it passes behind the medial malleolus and under the flexor retinaculum (laciniate ligament) in the medial ankle (the tarsal tunnel) (Figure 13-4).

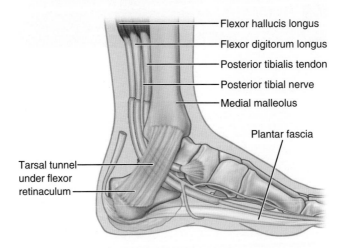

Figure 13-4 • Tarsal tunnel syndrome. (Reprinted from Anderson MK. *Foundations of Athletic Training*. Baltimore: Wolters Kluwer; 2012 with permission.)

- Pain, tightness, burning, numbness/tingling behind medial malleolus radiating along the arch and plantar aspect of foot including the heel occur.
- Pain usually worsens during standing or activity; in one-third of patients, the pain radiates proximally up the medial leg.
- Is relatively rare; seen in runners.

Treatment
- NSAIDs
- Physical therapy
- Kinesiology taping

Kinesiology Taping for Shin Splints and Tarsal Tunnel Syndrome
- Measure and cut a piece of tape from the lateral aspect of the calcaneus to the medial tibia below the knee.
- Measure and cut a second piece of tape that will go horizontally around calf, without overlapping.
- For the long piece of tape, dorsiflex and internally rotate the foot.
- Place 1 inch of tape on the lateral aspect of the foot, tape across the calcaneus and arch; then apply a 50% stretch and move up along the medial tibial region, covering the area of greatest pain.
- Attach the last 3 cm of tape with no stretch.
- Rub the tape to activate it.

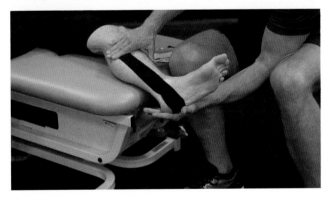

- For the small tape, rip it in the middle.
- Stretch it about 50%, and apply it perpendicular to the vertical strip over the area of greatest pain.
- Secure the lateral 3 cm on each end with no stretch; then rub to activate.

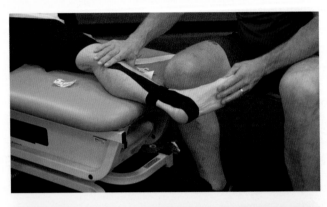

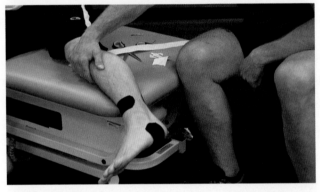

NAVICULAR FRACTURES

Diagnosis

- Common in runners; patients complain of gradual onset of vague dorsal midfoot pain associated with activity.

Examination

- The patient has tenderness on palpation over the dorsal aspect of the navicular bone (Figure 13-5).

Medial View

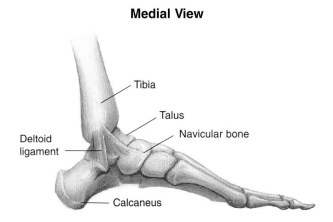

Figure 13-5 • Medial view of the foot showing the navicular bone. (Reprinted from Anatomical Chart Company with permission from Wolters Kluwer.)

- Pain can be elicited with passive eversion and active inversion.
- If x-ray is negative and suspicion is high, obtain a magnetic resonance image because x-ray has low sensitivity.

Treatment

- Treatment involves casting and non-weight bearing.

Treatment Summary

Soft Tissue Mobilization of Plantar Fascia

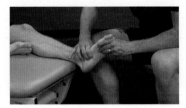
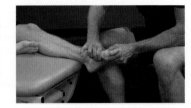

Active Release for Plantar Fasciitis

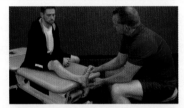
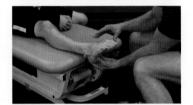

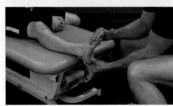

Navicular Sling

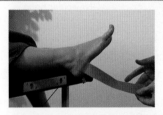
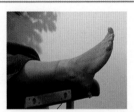

Spiral Tape for Inversion Sprain

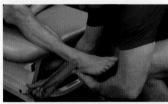
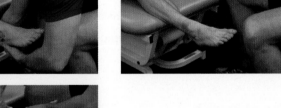

Calf Stretch for Achilles Tendonitis or Peroneal Tendonitis

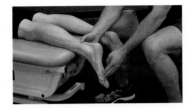 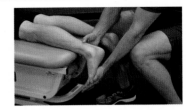

Trigger Point and Active Release for Achilles Tendonitis

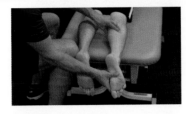

Kinesiology Taping for Achilles Tendonitis

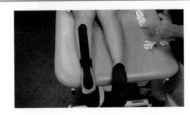

Kinesiology Taping for Lateral Ankle Symptoms

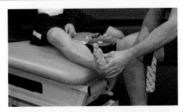 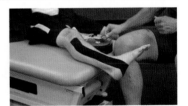

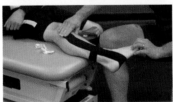

Shin Splint Anterior Tibialis Active Release

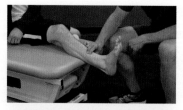
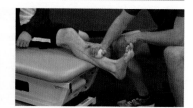

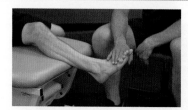

Shin Splint Anterior Tibialis Stretch/Relax

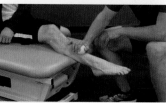

Kinesiology Taping for Medial Ankle Symptoms (Shin Splints and Tarsal Tunnel Syndrome)

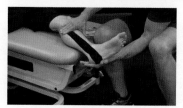
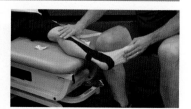

Sample Procedure Notes and Coding

Procedure:	**ICD-10-CM Diagnosis Codes:** Plantar Fasciitis: M25.57 Achilles Tendonitis: M76.6 Ankle Sprain: S93.40 Peroneal Tendonitis: M76.70 **CPT**: 97140 – Manual therapy techniques one or more regions	
	Minutes	Units Reported
	8-22	1
	23-37	2
	38-52	3
	53-67	4
	99070 – Supplies and Materials: provided by the qualified health care professional over and above those usually included with the office visit (list supplies/materials used)	
Informed Consent	After explaining the risks, benefits, and alternatives for the treatment, the patient gave verbal consent for the procedure	
Description of Procedure		
Outcomes/ Complications		
Instructions to Patient		
Time	Total time spent in **constant attendance** with the patient performing manual therapies: XX minutes	

Foam Roller

- Sit with your calf over a foam roller, supporting yourself with your arms (as shown).

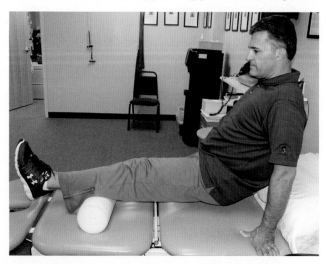

- Slowly roll the foam roller up and down along your calf muscles, rotating the leg to massage the calf from different angles.
- Identify areas of tightness and pain and adjust your force as necessary.
- Repeat 10 to 20 times.

Calf Stretch

- Try to perform this stretch before getting out of bed or after sitting for a long period.
- Sit with your knee straight and towel or stretching strap around the ball of the foot.

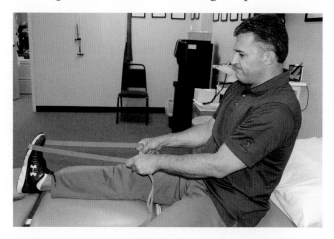

- Gently pull the towel until a stretch is felt in your calf. **DO NOT** just pull on your toes!
- Hold this position for 20 to 30 seconds and repeat three to five times.

Selected References

Fraser JJ, Corbett R, Donner C, Hertel J. Does manual therapy improve pain and function in patients with plantar fasciitis? A systematic review. *J Man Manip Ther*. 2018;26(2):55-65.

Mischke HH, Jayaseelan DJ, Sault JD, Emerson Kavchak AJ. The symptomatic and functional effects of manual physical therapy on plantar heel pain: a systematic review. *J Man Manip Ther*. 2017;25(1):3-10.

Figure Credits

INDEX

Note: Page numbers followed by "f" indicate figures, "t" indicate tables and "b" indicate boxes.

A

Abduction, pain/restriction with, 54–55, 54f–55f
Acetaminophen, 9
Achilles tendonitis
  arch support, 213
  calf stretch, 211, 211f, 223f
  diagnosis, 210, 210f
  foam roller, calf muscles, 213
  ice massage, 213
  kinesiology taping, 212, 212f, 223f
  physical examination, 210
  physical therapy, 213
  trigger point and active release for, 212, 212f, 223f
Adson sign, 73
Allopathic medicine, 4
Allopathic providers, 2
Angina, 71, 93
Anserine bursitis, 177
Anterior superior iliac spine (ASIS), 155, 164, 191
Apprehension testing, impingement syndrome, 53, 53f
Asthma, 16

B

Belly breaths. *See* Mindful breathing
Bilateral doorway stretch
  shoulder, 64, 64f
  upper crossed syndrome, 84, 84f

C

Carpal tunnel syndrome, 93, 99, 115
  flossing for, 102–103, 108f
  treatment for, 117f
  wrist mobilization, 108f
Cervical compression test, neck and upper back pain, 18, 18f
Cervical distraction, neck and upper back pain
  sitting position, 19, 19f
  supine, 20, 20f
Cervical radiculopathy, 93
Chest discomfort, acute
  costochondritis, 71. *See also* Costochondritis
  desk positioning, 91, 91f
    ball stretch, 89, 89f
    levator scapulae self-stretch, 89, 89f

    stretching strap, 86, 86f
    stretch with dowel, 85, 85f
    subscapularis stretching strap, 87–88, 87f–88f
  differential diagnosis, 71
  first rib syndrome and dysfunction, 72
    stretching strap exercises, 90, 90f
    treatment, 77, 77f, 79f
  history, 73
  physical examination, 73
  symptoms, 73
  treatment rules, 74
  upper crossed syndrome, 71, 72f. *See also* Upper crossed syndrome
Costochondritis
  costochondral junctions, 72
  kinesiology taping, 76, 76f, 78f
  lateral neck and trapezius, 75, 75f, 78f
  levator scapulae, 76, 76f, 78f
  pectoralis major stretch, 74, 74f, 78f
  pectoralis minor stretch, 75, 75f, 78f
  signs and symptoms, 72
Cubital tunnel syndrome, 93, 95
  "stop" gesture, 99
  treatment, 99, 99f
Current Procedure Terminology (CPT) procedure code, 11, 11t

D

Documentation
  "constant attendance," 12
  follow-up/interval visit, 12
  informed consent, 12
  initial visit, 12
  kinesiology tape, 13
  procedure note, 12
  requirements, 11

E

Elbow pain
  desk positioning, 116, 116f
  differential diagnosis, 93
  epicondylitis strap, 117, 118f
  forearm mobilization, 96, 96f, 107f
  lateral epicondylitis, 94
    instructions for, 117, 117f
    treatment for, 97, 97f, 107f

Elbow pain *(Continued)*
  medial epicondylitis, 94
    instructions for, 117, 117f
    treatment for, 98, 98f, 107f
  physical examination, 93, 94f
  pronator teres syndrome, 94
    physical examination, 94–95, 95f
    treatment for, 97, 97f
  treatment rules, 95
Electronic health record, 11
Empty can test, impingement syndromes, 51, 51f

F

Facet joint dysfunction, 119
First rib syndrome and dysfunction, 72
  stretching strap exercises, 90, 90f
  treatment, 77, 77f, 79f
Flexion abduction external rotation (FABER)
    test, 155–156, 155f–156f, 169, 169f
  adductor dysfunction, 173, 173f
  external rotators, 174, 174f
  hamstrings, piriformis, and gluteals,
    172, 172f
  iliotibial band stretch, side-lying, 175, 175f
Foot and ankle pain
  Achilles tendonitis. *See* Achilles tendonitis
  acute lateral ankle sprain. *See* Lateral ankle
    sprain, acute
  calf stretch, 226, 226f
  common causes, 202
  foam roller, 226, 226f
  navicular fractures, 221, 221f
  peroneal (lateral) tendonitis. *See* Peroneal
    (lateral) tendonitis
  plantar fasciitis. *See* Plantar fasciitis
  shin splints. *See* Shin splints
  tarsal tunnel syndrome. *See* Tarsal tunnel
    syndrome
  uncommon causes, 202

G

Gluteus bridge, 198, 198f
  extension bias, 148–149, 148f–149f
Golfer's elbow, 94. *See also* Medial epicondylitis

H

Hamstring bridge, 197, 197f
Hamstring stretch, 125–126, 125f–126f, 138f,
  144, 144f
  knee pain, 200, 200f
Hawkins test, impingement syndromes, 52, 52f
Headaches, 4, 16
Hip adductor, 152
  dysfunction, 173, 173f, 177, 200, 200f

external rotation adductor stretch,
    164– 165, 164f, 167f, 174, 174f
  reciprocal inhibition, 164, 164f, 167f
Hip extensor dysfunction, 152
Hip flexor stretches, 129, 129f, 139f, 144, 144f,
  148, 148f
  anterior hip pain, 159–160, 159f–160f, 166f
  patellofemoral syndrome, 181, 181f, 193f
Hip flexor tightness
  bridges, 170, 170f–171f
  lying hip stretch, 170f
  patellofemoral syndrome, 182, 193f
  reciprocal inhibition, 160, 160f, 166f
    patellofemoral syndrome, 182, 193f
Hypertension, 4

I

Iliopsoas spasm, 155
Iliotibial (IT) band syndrome, 152
  hold/relax for, 163, 163f, 167f
  Noble compression test, 161, 161f–162f
  Ober test, 162–163, 162f–163f
  stretch, 175, 175f
Infraspinatus and teres minor, 56–57, 56f–57f
Internal rotation, pain/restriction with, 57–58,
  57f–58f
International Classification of Diseases, Tenth
  Revision, Clinical Modification
  (ICD-10-CM) codes, 11

K

Kinesiology tape (K-Taping), 6, 9f
  achilles tendonitis, 212, 212f
  application, 10
  costochondritis, 76, 76f, 78f
  iliotibial (IT) band syndrome, 187–188,
    187f, 194f
  low back pain, acute, 136–137, 136f–137f,
    141f
  medial ankle pain, 219–220, 219f–220f
  neck support, 28, 28f, 33f
  patellar tendonitis/jumper knee, 182–183,
    182f–183f, 193f
  peroneal (lateral) tendonitis, 214–215,
    214f–216f
  postural support, 29–30, 29f–30f, 34f
  shoulder, 58, 58f
  tarsal tunnel syndrome, 219–220, 219f–220f
  upper back support, 30–31, 30f–31f, 34f
  upper crossed syndrome, 76, 76f, 78f
  usage, 9
  wrist pain
    lateral epicondylitis, 103–104,
      103f–104f, 108f

medial epicondylitis, 104–105,
104f–105f, 108f
pronator teres syndrome, 105–106,
105f–106f, 109f
Knee pain
acute
differential diagnosis, 178
without trauma, 178
adductor dysfunction, 200, 200f
differential diagnosis, 177
glute bridge, 198, 198f
hamstring bridge, 197, 197f
hamstring stretch, 200, 200f
injuries and dysfunctions, 177, 177f
lateral knee pain, 178
iliotibial band friction syndrome. See
Iliotibial (IT) band syndrome
with little/no edema, 178
medial knee pain, 179
external rotation adductor stretch, 191,
191f, 194f
kinesiology taping, anserine bursitis,
191–192, 192f, 195f
physical examination, 189, 189f
symptoms, 189
treatment, 189–190, 190f
normal vs. lost concavities, 178, 178f
patellar tendonitis/jumper knee
diagnosis, 180
kinesiology taping, 182–183, 182f–183f,
193f
patellofemoral syndrome
diagnosis, 180
hip flexor stretches, 181, 181f, 193f
hip flexor tightness, reciprocal inhibition,
182, 193f
quadriceps stretch, 198, 198f
quad sets, 199, 199f
with swelling, 178

L

Lateral ankle sprain, acute
diagnosis, 207
fracture locations, 207, 208f
spiral tape for, 209, 209f, 222f
Lateral epicondylitis, 93–94
instructions for, 117, 117f
kinesiology taping, 103–104, 103f–104f, 108f
treatment for, 97, 97f
Lateral neck and trapezius
costochondritis, 75, 75f, 78f
neck and upper back pain, 23, 23f, 32f
shoulder, 57, 57f
upper crossed syndrome, 75, 75f, 78f

Leg, upper and hip
adductor dysfunction, 173, 173f
external rotation adductor stretch, 164–
165, 164f, 167f, 174, 174f
reciprocal inhibition, 164, 164f, 167f
anterior hip pain, hip flexor stretches,
159–160, 159f–160f, 166f
differential diagnosis, 152
flexion abduction external rotation (FABER),
155–156, 155f–156f, 169, 169f
hip complex muscles, 152, 154f
hip flexor tightness
bridges, 170, 170f–171f
lying hip stretch, 170f
reciprocal inhibition, 160, 160f, 166f
iliac crest height, 153, 153f
iliotibial (IT) band dysfunction. See Iliotibial
(IT) band syndrome
palpation, 156
piriformis, 158, 158f, 166f
posterior leg pain, 166f
hamstrings, piriformis, gluteals, 157, 157f,
172, 172f
reciprocal inhibition, 159, 159f, 166f
treatment rules, 156
Levator scapulae, 23–24, 24f, 32f
costochondritis, 76, 76f, 78f
self stretch, 45, 45f
acute chest discomfort, 89, 89f
upper crossed syndrome, 76, 76f, 78f
Locked facet joint, 16
Low back pain, acute
extension bias, 119, 121, 121f
flexion bias, 119, 121, 121f
hip muscles, 120, 120f
joint mobilization, 120
kinesiology taping, 136–137, 136f–137f, 141f
piriformis syndrome, 132, 132f. See also
Piriformis syndrome
quadratus lumborum
reciprocal inhibition procedure, sitting
stretch, 130, 130f, 140f
self stretch, 150
side-lying stretch, 130–131, 130f–131f, 140f
range-of-motion (ROM) testing,
120, 122, 122f
rule out conditions, 121b
stability, 119, 119f
treatment, 120, 123
Low back pain, extension bias
gluteus bridge, 148–149, 148f–149f
hip flexor stretch, 129, 129f, 139f, 144, 144f,
148, 148f
leg pull, 128, 128f, 139f

Low back pain, extension bias *(Continued)*
    lumbar glide, 126–127, 126f–127f, 139f
    prone rectus femoris, 128, 128f, 139f
    psoas stretch, 128, 128f, 139f
    quadriceps, 148–149, 148f–149f
    rectus femoris stretch, 127–128, 127f, 139f
    sleeping positioning, 149
    stretching strap/dowel stretch, 147, 148f
    supine psoas, 127–128, 127f, 139f
    techniques, 126
    treatment, 126
Low back pain, flexion bias
    assisted posterior pelvic tilt, 124, 124f, 138f
    cannonball, 123, 123f–124f, 138f
    Hamstring stretch, 125–126, 125f–128f, 138f,
        144, 144f
    isometric posterior pelvic tilt, 145, 145f
    resting stretch, 146, 146f
    straight-leg raise, traction, 125, 125f, 138f
    stretching strap/dowel, 143–144, 143f–144f
    techniques, 123
    treatment, 123
Lumbar radiculopathies, 119

M

Manual medicine, 2–4
    application, 5
    benefits, 5
    billing, 11
    Current Procedure Terminology
        (CPT) procedure code, 11
        time based, 11t
    documentation
        "constant attendance," 12
        follow-up/interval visit, 12
        informed consent, 12
        initial visit, 12
        kinesiology tape, 13
        procedure note, 12
        requirements, 11
Medial ankle pain
    diagnosis, 218–219, 218f
    kinesiology taping, 219–220, 219f–220f, 224f
    treatment, 219
Medial epicondylitis, 93–94
    instructions for, 117, 117f
    kinesiology taping, 104–105, 104f–105f, 108f
    treatment for, 98, 98f
Medial tibial stress syndrome. *See* Shin splints
Meditation, 7
Methicillin-resistant *Staphylococcus aureus*, 2
Mid-back stretches
    dowel stretch, 44, 44f
    floor stretch, 43, 43f

levator scapulae self stretch, 45, 45f
Mimic angina, 16
Mindful breathing, 7
    clinical benefits, 8
    method for, 7
Mindfulness, 7
Muscle energy techniques, 5
Muscle spasm/torticollis, 16
Myofascial release, 4

N

Navicular fractures, 221, 221f
Neck and upper back pain
    acute pain, 16
    cervical compression test, 18, 18f
    cervical distraction
        sitting position, 19, 19f
        supine, 20, 20f
    chronic neck strain, 16
    differential diagnosis, 16
    doorway stretch, 42, 42f
    history, 16
    kinesiology taping
        neck support, 28, 28f, 33f
        postural support, 29–30, 29f–30f, 34f
        upper back support, 30–31, 30f–31f, 34f
    manual therapy
        anterior neck and upper back, 22–23, 23f,
            32f
        lateral neck and trapezius, 23, 23f, 32f
        levator scapulae, 23–24, 24f, 32f
        quadratus lumborum, upper and mid back,
            26, 26f, 33f
        rhomboids, medial upper back, 24–25,
            24f–25f, 33f
        strain/counterstain, 27, 27f, 33f
        trunk rotators, 25–26, 25f–26f, 33f
    mid-back stretches
        dowel stretch, 44, 44f
        floor stretch, 43, 43f
        levator scapulae self stretch, 45, 45f
    mobilization
        chin tuck, 22, 22f, 37, 37f
        tennis/softball, 38, 38f
        towel/strap stretching, 21, 21f–22f, 32f, 36,
            36f–37f
    physical examination
        muscle spasm and trigger points, 17–18, 17f
        postural assessment, 17
        range of motion (ROM), 17
    postural correction, 20
    rhomboid stretches
        door-frame stretch, 46–47, 46f–47f
        and middle trapezius self stretch, 48, 48f

scalenes stretch, 38–39, 38f–39f
spurling test, 19, 19f
treatment rules, 20
upper trapezius ball self massage, 41, 41f
wall stretch, 40, 40f
Neer test, impingement syndromes, 52, 52f
Noble compression test, 161, 161f–162f,
    184–185, 184f–185f
Nonsteroidal anti-inflammatory drugs
    (NSAIDs), 9, 206

O

Ober test, 162–163, 162f–163f, 186, 186f
"One-Second Mindfulness" method, 8
Osteoarthritis, 2, 99
    cervical spine, 16
Osteopathic providers, 2
Osteopathy, 4
Ottawa rules, 207

P

Patellar compression test, 180
Patellar tendonitis/jumper knee, 177
    diagnosis, 180
    kinesiology taping, 182–183, 182f–183f, 193f
Patellofemoral syndrome, 177
    diagnosis, 180
    hip flexor stretches, 181, 181f, 193f
    hip flexor tightness, reciprocal inhibition,
        182, 193f
Patrick testing, 155–156, 155f–156f
Pectoralis/anterior capsule stretch, 64, 64f
    acute chest discomfort, 84, 84f
Pectoralis major stretch
    costochondritis, 74, 74f, 78f
    upper crossed syndrome, 74, 74f, 78f
Pectoralis minor stretch
    costochondritis, 75, 75f, 78f
    upper crossed syndrome, 75, 75f, 78f
Pelvic tilt, posterior, 145, 145f
Peroneal (lateral) tendonitis
    arch support taping, 214
    calf stretch, 214, 214f
    diagnosis, 213
    distal fibula, 213, 213f
    foam roller, calf muscles, 214
    ice massage, 214
    kinesiology taping, 214–215, 214f–216f, 223f
    physical therapy, 214
Physical rehabilitation, 2
PIR. *See* Post isometric relaxation (PIR)
Piriformis dysfunction, 152
    upper leg and hip, 158, 158f
Piriformis muscle spasm, 119

Piriformis syndrome
    prone piriformis release, 135, 135f, 141f
    radiculopathy and sciatica, 132
    side-lying stretch, 132–133, 132f–133f, 140f
    stretch, 145, 144f
    supine stretch, 133–134, 133f–134f, 140f
Plantar fasciitis
    active release for, 204–205, 204f–205f, 222f
    diagnosis, 202
    foam roller/tennis ball, 206
    navicular sling for, 205–206, 205f–206f,
        222f
    night splints, 206
    orthotics straps, 206
    plantar fasciitis straps, 206
    self-massage, 206
    soft tissue mobilization, 202, 203f, 222f
    tibialis anterior and posterior mobilization,
        203, 203f–204f
    weight reduction, 206
Positional release therapy, 4
Post isometric relaxation (PIR), 5
Pronator teres syndrome, 93–94
    kinesiology taping, 105–106, 105f–106f, 109f
    physical examination
        cubital tunnel syndrome, 95
        tests for, 94, 95f
        treatment, 97, 97f
Prone piriformis release, 135, 135f, 141f
Prone rectus femoris, 128, 128f, 139f
Proprioceptive neuromuscular facilitation
    (PNF). *See* Post isometric relaxation
    (PIR)
Psoas stretch, 128, 128f, 139f
Pulmonary embolism, 71

Q

Quadratus lumborum
    reciprocal inhibition procedure, sitting
        stretch, 130, 130f, 140f
    self stretch, 150
    side-lying stretch, 130–131, 130f–131f, 140f
    upper and mid back pain, 26, 26f, 33f
Quadriceps dysfunction, 180
Quadriceps stretch, 198, 198f
Quad sets, 199, 199f

R

Randomized controlled trials, 5, 9
Reciprocal inhibition (RI), 5
    adductor dysfunction, 164, 164f, 167f
    hip flexor tightness, 160, 160f
    posterior leg pain, 159, 159f
    procedure, sitting stretch, 130, 130f, 140f

Rectus femoris stretch, 127–128, 127f, 139f
Referred pain, 152
Rehabilitation, 5–6, 10
Resting stretch, flexion bias, 146, 146f
Restrictive barrier, 5
Rhomboids stretches, 24–25, 24f–25f, 33f
  door-frame stretch
    neck and upper back pain, 46–47, 46f–47f
    shoulder, 65, 65f
  and middle trapezius self stretch
    neck and upper back pain, 48, 48f
    and shoulder, 69, 69f
RI. *See* Reciprocal inhibition (RI)
Rotator cuff tendonitis. *See* Impingement
    syndrome

S
Sacroiliac joint dysfunction, 155
Scalenes stretch, 38–39, 38f–39f
Shin splints
  anterior tibialis active release, 217, 217f, 224f
  anterior tibialis stretch/relax, 218, 218f, 224f
  diagnosis, 216
  physical examination, 216
Shoulder
  bilateral doorway stretch, 64, 64f
  differential diagnosis, 51
  impingement, 93
  impingement syndromes, 50. *See also*
      Impingement syndromes
  infraspinatus and teres minor, 56–57, 56f–57f
  isometric scapular engagement, 62, 62f
  kinesiology taping, 58, 58f
  lateral neck and trapezius, 57, 57f
  mobilization with softball, 60, 60f
  muscle-tendon structures, 50
  physical therapy program, 50
  range of motion, 61, 61f
  rhomboids stretches
    door-frame stretch, 65, 65f
    and middle trapezius self- stretch, 69, 69f
  rotator cuff anatomy, 50, 50f
  self-stretch, 63, 63f
  subscapularis
    stretches, 66, 66f
    stretching strap, 67–68, 67f–68f
    treatment, 55–56, 55f–56f
  supraspinatus treatment, 54–55, 54f–55f
  trauma-related shoulder pain, 50
  treatment rules, 53
Shoulder impingement syndromes, 2
  active range of motion, 51
  empty can test, 51, 51f

Hawkins test, 52, 52f
history, 51
joint laxity/subluxation/dislocation testing,
    53, 53f
Neer test, 52, 52f
passive range of motion, 51
Shoulder pain/restriction with external
    rotation, 55–56, 55f–56f
Spurling test, neck and upper back pain,
    19, 19f
Subscapularis
  dysfunction, 16
  stretching strap, acute chest discomfort,
    87–88, 87f–88f

T
Tarsal tunnel syndrome
  diagnosis, 218–219, 218f
  kinesiology taping, 219–220, 219f–220f, 224f
  treatment, 219
Tender points formation, 4
Tennis elbow, 94. *See also* Lateral epicondylitis
Thoracic outlet syndrome, 72–73
Tight hip extensor, sciatica, 158, 158f
Trigger points, 12
Trunk rotators, upper back pain, 25–26,
    25f–26f, 33f

U
Ulnar nerve impingement. *See* Cubital tunnel
    syndrome
Upper back stretches
  doorway stretch, 42, 42f
  upper trapezius ball self massage, 41, 41f
  wall stretch, 40, 40f
Upper crossed syndrome
  bilateral doorway stretch, 84, 84f
  isometric scapular engagement, 82, 82f
  kinesiology taping, 76, 76f, 78f
  lateral neck and trapezius, 75, 75f, 78f
  levator scapulae, 76, 76f, 78f
  pectoralis major stretch, 74, 74f, 78f
  pectoralis minor stretch, 75, 75f, 78f
  range of motion, 81, 81f
  wall and neck stretch, 83, 83f

W
Whiplash, 16
Wrist pain
  anatomy, 99, 100f
  carpal tunnel syndrome, 99, 115
    flossing for, 102–103, 108f
    treatment for, 107f

differential diagnosis, 99
kinesiology taping
  lateral epicondylitis, 103–104, 103f–104f,
    108f
  medial epicondylitis, 104–105, 104f–105f,
    108f
  pronator teres syndrome, 105–106,
    105f–106f, 109f

mobilization, 100–101, 100f–101f
  traction with, flexion/extension, 101–102,
    102f, 108f
range of motion (ROM), 111, 111f
resisted flexion and extension, 113–114,
  113f–114f
traction, 112, 112f
Wrist sprain, differential diagnosis, 99